Emergency Management in Health Care

An All-Hazards Approach

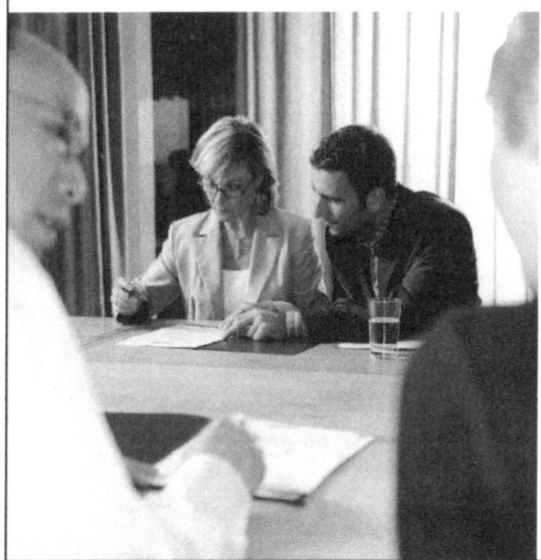

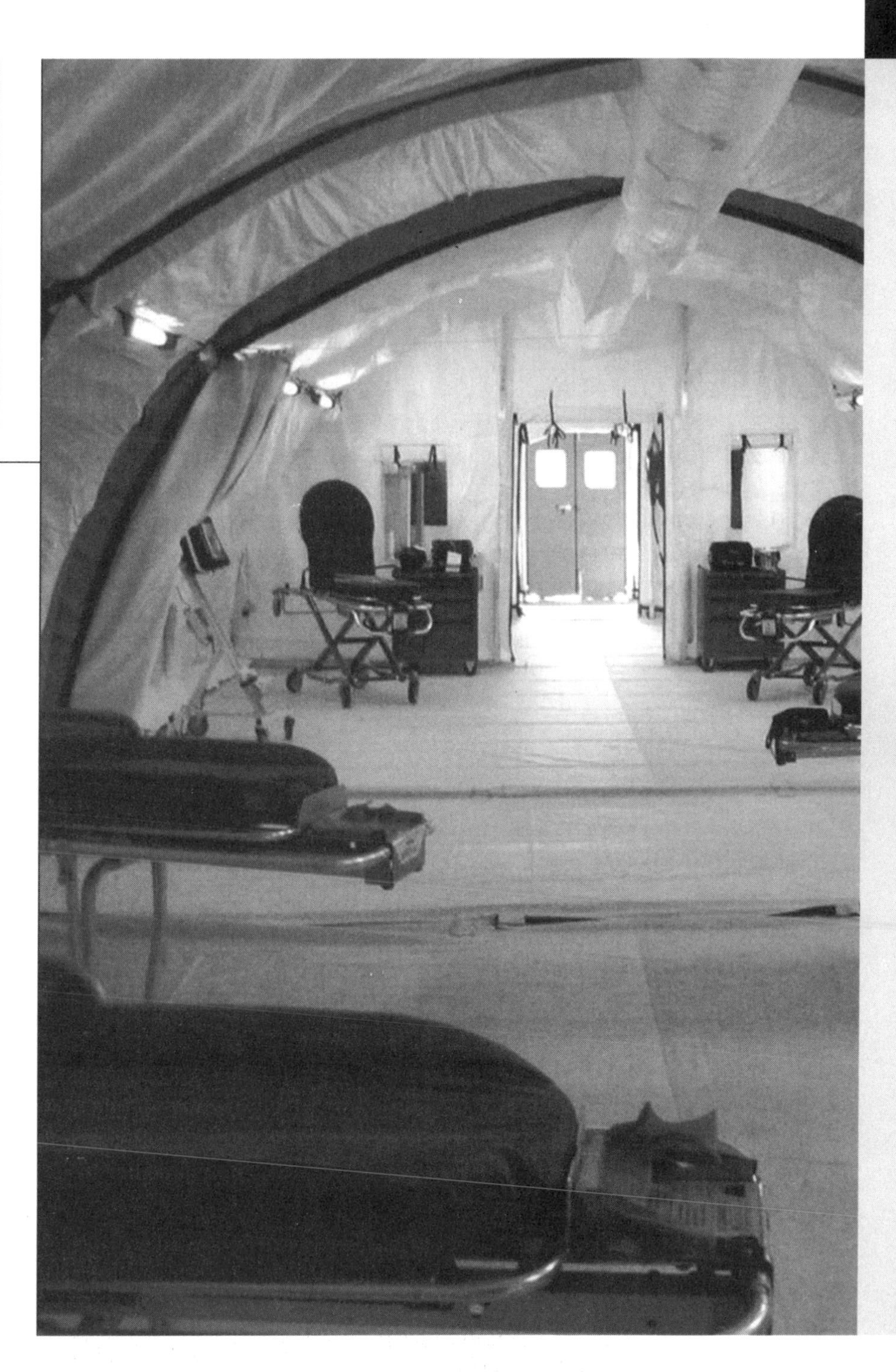

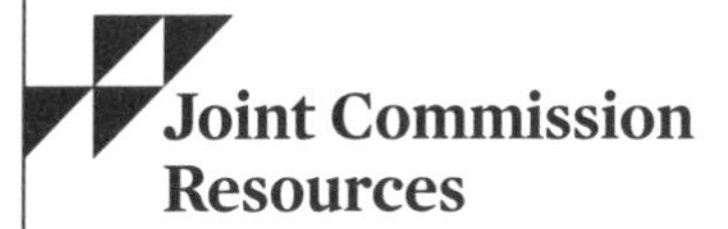

Joint Commission Resources

Senior Editor: Robert A. Porché, Jr.
Project Manager: Andrew Bernotas
Manager, Publications: Victoria Smith
Associate Director, Production: Johanna Harris
Associate Director, Editorial Development: Diane Bell
Executive Director: Catherine Chopp Hinckley, Ph.D.
Vice President, Learning: Charles Macfarlane, F.A.C.H.E.
Joint Commission/JCR Reviewers: Pat Adamski, Lynne Bergero, John Fishbeck, Jerry Gervais, Kristine Miller, George Mills, Ken Peterson, Charles "Skip" Wilson

Joint Commission Resources Mission
The mission of Joint Commission Resources is to continuously improve the safety and quality of care in the United States and in the international community through the provision of education and consultation services and international accreditation.

Joint Commission Resources educational programs and publications support, but are separate from, the accreditation activities of The Joint Commission. Attendees at Joint Commission Resources educational programs and purchasers of Joint Commission Resources publications receive no special consideration or treatment in, or confidential information about, the accreditation process.

Printed in the U.S.A. 5 4 3 2 1

ISBN: 978-1-59940-185-0
Library of Congress Control Number: 2008921936

For more information about Joint Commission Resources, please visit http://www.jcrinc.com.

Contents

Introduction

- The September 11, 2001, terrorist attacks
- The blackout of 2003
- A 2004 hurricane season that pounded Florida
- Hurricanes Katrina and Rita that struck the Gulf Coast in 2005
- A Hawaiian earthquake
- The 2007 bridge collapse in Minnesota
- A series of at least 14 tornadoes that whipped across Georgia in 2007

This series of highly visible events has demonstrated the pressing need for enhanced emergency management that will allow health care organizations to adequately respond to incidents that create mass casualties. Whether the emergency results from nature (such as hurricanes, earthquakes, floods, blizzards, or tornadoes), from unintentional occurrences (such as train or plane accidents; power failures; or accidents involving nuclear, biological, or chemical contamination), or from intentional terrorist attacks (such as biological or chemical attacks or massive bombings), adequate preparation by health care organizations is critical to the nation as a whole and to the communities in which the organizations operate. Communities turn to health care organizations to provide medical care to those injured following an emergency or a disaster. Often, however, the organizations themselves and their staffs are also victims of the disaster. Organizations must be prepared to provide care to those injured in the community while at the same time be able to protect their own staff and facilities.

Recent disasters have also made it clear that it is not enough for health care organizations to plan for individual emergency events. Instead, organizations committed to serving their communities must demonstrate the ability to respond to combinations of escalating events. With this in mind, The Joint Commission revised its emergency management standards for hospitals, critical access hospitals, and Medicare- and Medicaid-based long term care organizations in 2008. Specifically, the standard that requires organizations to address emergency management was broadened into eight new standards that became effective January 1, 2008.

The revised standards are designed to help health care organizations cope with a major destructive incident that could present an overwhelming number of patients and that could affect or disrupt their own environments of care and the lives in surrounding communities. Since September 11, 2001, much media attention has focused on health care organizations' preparedness to respond to mass casualty incidents. Public health experts, industry officials, and the Joint Commission's work in this area all indicate that health care organizations need practical guidance to prepare for, respond to, and recover from emergencies.

Using Lessons Learned

In formulating the revised emergency management standards, The Joint Commission sought input from health care organizations affected by disasters, engaged emergency management experts, served on national emergency management panels, and reviewed current literature on emergency management. From these studies, The Joint Commission concluded that it is not sufficient to require health care organizations to plan for a single event; rather, they should be able to demonstrate sufficient flexibility to respond effectively to combinations of escalating events.

Since the inception of the Joint Commission's accreditation programs for health care organizations, compliance with the Joint Commission emergency management standards has helped to ensure organization readiness to respond to both internal and external emergencies. Given recent national experience with natural and man-made disasters, The Joint Commission is committed to reinforcing a comprehensive approach, recommended through the emergency management planning standards (*see* Chapters 1 through 10).

What's New

Specific revisions to the emergency management standards (effective January 1, 2008) include the following:

- The previous single emergency management–related standard has been replaced by a series of stand-alone emergency management standards. Although some of the elements of performance in this series of standards are new, many are existing expectations that have been relocated or moderately edited. The edits were made to provide clear guidance to organizations in their emergency management planning efforts.
- The addition of requirements for managing the following six critical areas regardless of the cause(s) of an emergency situation:
  1. Communication
  2. Resources and assets
  3. Safety and security
  4. Staff responsibilities
  5. Utilities management
  6. Patient clinical and support activities
- The addition of requirements for evaluating the performance of these six critical areas during planned exercises
- The addition of a requirement for conducting at least one exercise per year to evaluate how effectively the organization performs when it cannot be supported by the local community

The revisions to the emergency management standards reflect an "all-hazards" approach that permits flexible and effective responses. The standards emphasize a scalable approach that can help manage the variety, intensity, and duration of the disasters that can affect a single organization, multiple organizations, or an entire community. The revised standards also promote the importance of planning and testing response plans for emergencies during conditions when the local community cannot support the health care organization.

Overview of Contents

Emergency Management in Health Care: An All-Hazards Approach has been developed as a practical guide to help health care organizations plan for managing the critical areas of emergency response by assessing their needs and preparing staff to respond to events most likely to occur, regardless of the cause(s) of the emergency situation. This publication is directed to facility managers, performance improvement coordinators, survey coordinators, medical staff directors, directors of nursing, emergency department staff, safety managers and staff, and risk managers in health care organizations. The book will also be of interest to consultants and medical librarians.

This book guides hospitals, critical access hospitals, and long term care organizations in planning for the management of the six crucial areas of emergency response and encourages and enables them to assess their needs and prepare staff to respond to events that are likely to occur. With a sound understanding of and specific plans for their responses to these six areas, organizations can develop an all-hazards approach that supports a level of preparedness sufficient to address a range of emergencies. Specifically, the book is arranged as follows:

- Chapter 1 provides an overview of the six critical functions of emergency management.
- Chapter 2 provides guidance on addressing emergency management planning issues that are crucial to establishing a comprehensive emergency management strategy.
- Chapter 3 addresses the development of an emergency operations plan.
- Chapter 4 guides organizations in establishing emergency communications strategies, both within and outside the organization.
- Chapter 5 addresses how to establish strategies for managing resources and assets that are necessary to adequately respond to an emergency.
- Chapter 6 examines how to manage the safety and security of patients, which is the primary responsibility of an organization during an emergency.
- Chapter 7 provides guidance for defining and managing staff roles and responsibilities during an emergency that could require adapting roles as new demands arise. This chapter also addresses preparation and response strategies for the human and organization impact of emergencies.
- Chapter 8 addresses strategies to manage essential utilities such as electricity, water, fuel, ventilation, and so forth.

- Chapter 9 covers how to have clear and reasonable plans in place that address the clinical and other needs of patients and residents when an organization's resources are taxed by an emergency.
- Chapter 10 describes how organizations can test their emergency operation plans.

Throughout the book, there are case examples of effective emergency management plans and responses of health care organizations that have dealt with real-life emergencies.

Use of This Publication

The examples, checklists, tips, and documents included in this book come from a wide range of sources and address numerous types of disasters. Some of the information might be relevant to your organization or program; some might not. Staff in each organization must create emergency management processes, policies, and documents that are best suited to the organization's specific needs based on its hazard vulnerability analysis, as described in Chapter 2. You should use the information included here as a reference and starting point and adapt it to meet your organization's specific needs for an all-hazards emergency operations plan.

Note: This publication is designed to provide accurate and authoritative information regarding emergency management planning. Every attempt has been made to ensure accuracy at the time of publication; however, please note that laws, regulations, and standards are subject to change. Also note that some of the examples in this publication are specific to the laws and regulations of the organization's locality. The information and examples in this publication are provided with the understanding that the publisher is not engaged in providing medical, legal, or other professional advice. If any such assistance is desired, the services of a competent professional person should be sought.

Terminology and Taxonomy

Some clarification on the use of the term *emergency* throughout this book is in order. The Joint Commission's environment of care standards for accredited critical access hospitals, hospitals, and long term care organizations require an emergency operations plan that describes the organization's approach to responding to emergencies within the organization or in its community that would suddenly and significantly affect the need for the organization's services or its ability to provide those services. In this context, an emergency is a natural, unintentional, or intentional incident that significantly disrupts the environment of care (for example, damage to the organization's building[s] and grounds due to severe winds, storms, or earthquakes). An emergency is also an incident that significantly disrupts care and treatment (for example, loss of utilities, such as power, water, or telephones, due to floods, civil disturbances, accidents, or emergencies within the organization or its community) or results in sudden, significantly changed, or increased demands for the organization's services (for example, bioterrorist attack, building collapse, or plane crash in the organization's community).

Beyond The Joint Commission, emergencies have been classified in many different ways. Some systems, particularly in the health care literature, define two categories: internal emergencies and external emergencies. Internal emergencies are those that damage an organization's infrastructure (for example, a power failure or roof collapse), making it difficult, if not impossible, to provide care and services. External emergencies are those that occur beyond the organization's walls and that threaten to overwhelm the organization with a greatly increased patient volume. External and internal emergencies can happen simultaneously, such as when an earthquake damages a health care facility and results in large-scale casualties in the community.

Some classification systems use three categories: natural disasters (such as floods and hurricanes), technological disasters (such as transportation accidents, structural collapses, and chemical releases), and sociological and public health disasters (such as civil disturbances, arson, bombing, and bioterrorism). Others define the three categories a bit differently: natural disasters (such as tornadoes, forest fires, and earthquakes), unintentional disasters (such as airplane or other mass transportations accidents or nuclear accidents), and intentional disasters (such as biological or chemical attacks, massive explosions, or bombings).

Finally, throughout the publication, the words *patient* and *resident* are used interchangeably to describe the care recipient, consumer, individual receiving care, or the person who actually receives health care services.

Acknowledgments

We wish to express our appreciation to those members of The Joint Commission and Joint Commission Resources staff who reviewed the manuscript and/or advised in its development, including Pat Adamski, Ken Peterson, John Fishbeck, Charles "Skip" Wilson, George Mills, Lynne Bergero, Kristine Miller, Victoria Smith, and Diane Bell. We would particularly like to thank Jerry Gervais, an associate director with the Joint Commission's Standards Interpretation Group, for his invaluable advice and assistance. We are also deeply indebted to our writer, Janet McIntyre, for her careful attention to detail and her consummate professionalism.

Chapter 1

The Six Critical Functions of Emergency Management

Earthquakes, tornadoes, heat waves, floods, oil spills, fires, nuclear accidents, dirty bombs, pandemic flu, hurricanes, blackouts, blizzards. The list of disasters is endless—and continues to grow. On average, disasters cause 185 deaths per day. The loss of human life; the physical and environmental damages; the disruption to school, homes, business, and productivity; and the financial impact can be devastating to any country, city, and/or town.

Billions of people in more than a hundred countries will be exposed over the course of their lives to at least one earthquake, cyclone, flood, or drought.[1] But the impact of these, and many disasters, can be sharply reduced if we make an effort to assess risk, to develop and test contingency plans, and to respond to a disaster before it happens, rather than after the damage has been done. The message is clear, regardless of the disaster—similar considerations can provide good planning for most events encountered. The bottom line is that all health care organizations can and should be prepared to operate in a state of constant readiness.

The Joint Commission's emergency management standards are designed to help organizations achieve this readiness. Organizations that plan for managing six critical areas of emergency response are better able to asses their needs and prepare staff to respond to events most likely to occur, regardless of the causes of the emergency situation. The six critical areas are communication, resources and supplies, security, staff responsibilities, utilities management, and patient care.

The Joint Commission identified these six areas by categorizing the lessons learned from organizations interviewed following large-scale disasters, such as the 2004 hurricanes in Florida and Hurricanes Katrina and Rita in 2005. When organizations have a sound understanding of their response to these critical areas of emergency management, they have developed an "all-haz-

Revisions to Emergency Management Standards

- Standard EC.4.10 replaced by nine emergency management standards
- Became effective January 1, 2008
- Effective for hospitals, critical access hospitals, long term care organizations, Medicare-/Medicaid-based long term care programs

Revised Standards Versus Previous Standards

- All 21 elements of performance (EPs) from former Standard EC.4.10 still present in revised standards
- 30-plus additional EPs incorporated into emergency management standards

Rationale for Change

The revised standards are designed to accomplish the following:

- Emphasize a scalable approach to manage the variety, intensity, and duration of the disasters that can affect a single organization, multiple organizations, an entire community, or region
- Stress the importance of planning and testing response plans for emergencies during conditions when the local community cannot support the health care organization

ards" approach that supports a level of preparedness sufficient to address a range of emergencies, regardless of the cause. This chapter briefly describes the six critical areas of emergency management, which are discussed individually and in combination with other requirements in subsequent chapters of this book.

Communication

In the event that community infrastructure is damaged and/or an organization's power or facilities experience debilitation, communication pathways, whether dependent on fiber-optic cables, electricity, satellite, or other conduits, are likely to fail. Organizations must develop a plan to maintain communication pathways both within the organization and to critical community resources. The Joint Commission's expectations related to communication are explored in Chapter 4.

Resources and Assets

A solid understanding of the scope and availability of an organization's resources and assets is as important, and perhaps more important, during an emergency than during times of normal operation. Materials and supplies and vendor and community services, as well as state and federal programs, are some of the essential resources that organizations must know how to access in times of crisis to ensure patient safety and sustain care, treatment, and services. Details regarding organizational planning for resources and assets during an emergency can be found in Chapter 5.

Safety and Security

The safety and security of patients is the prime responsibility of the organization during an emergency. As emergency situations develop and parameters of operability shift, organizations must provide safe and secure environments for their patients and staff. This concept is explored in Chapter 6 of this book.

Staff Responsibilities

One of the emergency management standards addresses staff responsibilities, which is one of the critical functions of emergency management. During an emergency, the probability that staff responsibilities will change is high. As new risks develop along with changing conditions, staff will need to adapt their roles to meet new demands on their abilities to care for patients. If staff cannot anticipate how they might be called to perform during an emergency, the likelihood increases that the organization will not sustain itself during an emergency. Chapter 7 addresses the issues surrounding defining and managing staff roles and responsibilities.

Utilities Management

An organization depends on the uninterrupted function of its utilities during an emergency. The supply of key utilities, such as power, potable water, ventilation, and fuel, must not be disrupted or adverse events could occur as a result. The details surrounding this requirement and the framework for managing this critical function are discussed in Chapter 8.

Patient Clinical and Support Activities

The clinical needs of patients during an emergency are of prime importance, according to one of the revised emergency management standards. The organization must have clear, reasonable plans to address the needs of patients during extreme conditions when the organization's infrastructure and resources are taxed. Chapter 9 examines the accreditation requirements associated with patient clinical and support activities.

Best Practices for Success[2]

The Joint Commission emergency management standards require organizations to take a holistic approach to managing an emergency—not only preparing for a coordinated response but anticipating problems and ensuring self-efficiency. Effective emergency management requires planning and preparation efforts and complete and total support from everyone in an organization—from leadership to front-line staff.

The Joint Commission's emergency management standards address a variety of issues, including the need for an emergency operations plan, which outlines the incident command system and designates roles and responsibilities during an emergency. In addition, the standards require organizations to address the six critical functions outlined in this chapter that can profoundly affect the outcome of an emergency: communication, resources and assets, safety and security, staff responsibilities, utilities management, and clinical and support activities. The following sections explore how organizations can meet the standards and their content.

Working with the Community

Preparing for an emergency cannot happen in a vacuum. "All [emergency management] planning should be done in the context of the community. You should know where your organization fits in a community response, including what your organization can offer as well as what you can expect in the way of help and mutual aid," says Jerry Gervais, C.H.F.M., C.H.S.P., associate director, Standards Interpretation Group, The Joint Commission. Effectively working with the community includes coordinating with local community emergency responders—such as the police department, fire department, and emergency medical technicians—the local public health department, and any regional or statewide emergency operations entities. "It is critical that your organization not only understand how the local, regional, and statewide emergency operations command systems function but also be an active member in those entities when appropriate. By having a seat at the table, you can ensure your organization's voice is heard and your needs are met," says Gervais.

In addition, it is important for organizations to use the same terminology as their local, regional, and state emergency operations commands with regard to emergency management so communication can be effective. This may involve using a recognized incident command system such as the Hospital Incident Command System (HICS) or the National Incident Management System (NIMS). (For more information on HICS and NIMS, *see* Chapter 3.)

Working with Other Health Care Organizations

To ensure a coordinated response to an emergency, health care organizations must also open up a dialogue with other health care organizations in the area. It is important to establish contact and build relationships before an emergency. "This may mean talking with direct competitors about how you can support each other during unplanned situations," says Gervais. "During an emergency, the organizations you compete with every day become your partners. By establishing a relationship *before* an emergency, you can ensure that partnership is solid and complete."

Tightening Relationships with Suppliers

Before an emergency, organizations should consider tightening up any relationships they have with suppliers and making sure those suppliers can deliver supplies during an emergency. This includes discussing with a supplier the ways the company will get supplies to the health care organization and how many other health care organizations the supplier has agreed to supply. "For example, if a supplier has only one route of delivery—let's say by truck via an access road—and that road is unusable during an emergency, an organization should have a contingency plan worked out with the supplier so that supplies are brought via another route," says Gervais. "Likewise, if a supplier has agreed to deliver supplies to four other hospitals in the area during an emergency, it is possible that supplier will be unable to fill all of its commitments. During an emergency is not the time to find out that your supplier has overcommitted. The organization should talk with both the supplier and other health care organizations in the area to determine the depth and breadth of the supply chain." It is also a prudent move to contact suppliers out of the local area or even out of state/region as a backup plan. Local suppliers might experience the same issues (flooding, lack of staff, loss of power, and so on) as your organization.

Addressing an Evacuation

One aspect of emergency management with which organizations often struggle is evacuation. According to the Joint Commission standards, an organization must set specific criteria that outline the time frame the organization is able to stay and effectively "weather" an emergency versus when it will close or evacuate. "If an organization chooses to stay, it must have plans to be self-sufficient for 96 hours. If this is not possible, then the organization should have plans in place to evacuate after a predetermined period," says Gervais. For example, an organization might determine that it can be self-sufficient during an emergency for 48 hours, after which point it will initiate evacuation procedures. However, the organization should also make sure that its evacuation plan can be supported 48 hours after the start of an emergency. If the organization begins evacuating at 48 hours and the rest of the community has evacuated after 12 hours, the health care organization may run into significant problems. Once again, the need for community coordination is paramount.

"To effectively evacuate your facility, you have to understand how the evacuation will unfold, including who will be evacuated first and how the evacuation will safely proceed," says Gervais. "You also must understand where you are going when you evacuate and what happens to patients when you get there." To effectively prepare for evacuation, organizations should determine who has the authority to call an evacuation and ensure that all the staff knows who that person is. Staff members should also know their roles and responsibilities when an evacuation is called. "Basically, organizations should define an evacuation process to follow and ensure everyone in the organization is clear on that process," says Gervais.

Organizations should also consider what to do when the emergency is over. They should define who has the authority to declare an emergency over and have a specific plan that addresses the financial, staff, and patient care aspects of recovery.

Case Example: Flooding Threatens Hospital's Utility Systems, Tests Emergency Management Plan

Our Lady of Lourdes Memorial Hospital sits close to the banks of the Susquehanna River in Binghamton, New York. Part of the Catholic health ministry known as Ascension Health, the hospital's main campus includes an ambulatory surgery center and a regional cancer center. In April 2005 the organization's leaders responded to predictions of a storm that could bring a 100-year flood to the area by quickly building an 8-foot berm near the river's edge. When that storm arrived, the berm held up. A little over a year later, it would be tested again, as would the hospital's emergency management plan.

In accordance with emergency management planning standards, the 8-foot berm was built to separate the river from the hospital's parking lot and prevent water from threatening the facility and its power plant. "With the berm in place and additional adjustments made to our emergency management plan, we felt well prepared to deal with the impact of that 2005 storm," says John O'Neil, CEO. "When it passed without incident, we felt even more comfortable that we were in good shape."

Still, O'Neil says, when you're providing care to patients in a facility that stands near a river that is fed by up to 9,000 tributaries, you never feel too comfortable. On June 27, 2006, the storm that sent rising waters into communities elsewhere across the East Coast also brought flooding to areas of Binghamton. "The first day, we could see the water rising, and by the next morning, it was 5 to 6 feet up the berm," O'Neil recalls. Also in accordance with emergency management standards, Our Lady of Lourdes immediately set up an incident command center and, with a watchful eye on the river, began to consider further measures.

Taking Proactive Precautions

In keeping with Joint Commission requirements, those measures included communicating with the county's emergency management center as well as informing neighboring hospitals of a situation that could worsen and that might even involve transferring patients to those facilities. The situation did worsen later that morning. Although the berm continued to hold back the Susquehanna, water began to come up through the underground sewers and sanitary systems and into the hospital's water system. "That means you don't have clean water," says O'Neil. "This is something we hadn't considered, but as soon as we became aware of it, we began an evacuation of the ground floor."

Attempting to lessen the severity of a potentially larger evacuation, which is also addressed in Joint Commission emergency management standards, staff at Our Lady of Lourdes transferred critical patients to one of the neighboring hospitals; they also transferred patients whose physical condition would hamper the speed and safety of a full-scale evacuation. The hospital also discharged 35 patients whose treatments had been completed.

"Any time you move critically ill patients, it poses some risk to their safety," says Joseph Cappiello, former vice president, Accreditation Field Operations, Joint Commission. "But because they were thinking ahead and drew on their knowledge to recognize the dangerous possibility of being trapped in the facility with critical patients and others who are difficult to move, the hospital's leaders stayed one step ahead of the situation," he says. "They took a proactive rather than a reactive approach, and that's what emergency management planning is all about."

(continued)

Case Example: Flooding Threatens Hospital's Utility Systems, Tests Emergency Management Plan, *continued*

Relying on a Team Effort Evacuation

The pumps that the hospital activated on the facility's ground floor—which housed the pharmacy, laboratory, and sterile processing unit—were little help against the continuing flow of water that soon jeopardized the hospital's electrical system. "In the afternoon, we shut down the power, terminated operations, and began evacuating our 90 remaining inpatients," says O'Neil. This action also corresponds with Joint Commission emergency management standards related to temporarily closing or evacuating the facility.

During the throes of the evacuation effort, a pregnant patient gave birth. The infant was delivered safely and, with the mother and the other patients, was transferred in a process that involved two other hospitals, an ambulance system, and even a city bus. "In working as quickly as possible, we not only secured ambulances, but we were able to reach a city official who made a bus available to us for transferring," says O'Neil. "The entire evacuation and transfer process of 90 inpatients took only two hours, and there were no patient injuries."

Considering Every Emergency Angle

When O'Neil and other leaders in the incident command center were overseeing the evacuation, they were also in touch with the state's health department to gain credential approval for some of their own staff to transfer to the neighboring hospitals along with their patients.

"Through communication with the two other hospitals that were lending support, we had realized that a full evacuation would push them beyond capacity," O'Neil says. "Our staff would need to follow our patients to those hospitals and provide continuity of care. While our licenses and other paperwork were up to date, we had to verify this procedure with the state."

The approval process was smooth, and continuity of care was provided on the inpatient side as well as in the emergency departments at the other hospitals. In fact, Our Lady of Lourdes moved its entire nursing administration into one of the hospitals for the next 10 days. That's how long it took demolition crews to clean and begin to restore the more than $19 million in damage caused to 100,000 square feet of the hospital's ground floor.

Communication Is the Key to Preparation

As the potential for evacuation emerged, and as evacuation became necessary, O'Neil says the hospital's staff kept patients well informed of the situation and the role they would play. "We were very prepared, and our staff and patients responded incredibly well. Our patients seemed more worried about us and all the issues we had to deal with and coordinate," he says. "But every decision we made focused on patient safety."

The hospital's foresight in communicating early on with neighboring hospitals and its collaboration with local ambulance services and with the state's health department, O'Neil says, reflects a culture dedicated to patient care and patient safety. "At every step, patient safety was the top priority." Cappiello concurs. "Hospitals are often viewed as shelters in the case of emergencies, but even the best-laid plans can't overcome an emergency that threatens a facility and its patients. This hospital resisted temptations to ride out the incident, to wait and see what would happen next. Instead, its leaders examined the realities before them and took action," he says. "That's an important lesson here."

(continued)

Case Example: Flooding Threatens Hospital's Utility Systems, Tests Emergency Management Plan, *continued*

According to O'Neil, this experience has helped the organization strengthen its relationships not only with other health care systems but also with its community. "That is proving significant in our continued planning efforts," he says. Renewed flood mitigation services also continued at Our Lady of Lourdes. The hospital installed valves and storm gates in its underground systems to help prevent water from seeping into its water supply. "While a permanent solution will take years," O'Neil says, "we're quite confident in our emergency planning process and our capability to provide our patients with safe care."

Source: Reprinted from Joint Commission Resources: Come high water. *Environment of Care News* 10:2, Feb. 2007.

References

1. Joint Commission Resources: *Preparing for the Unknown: "Are You Ready?" Emergency Preparedness Conference.* http://www.jcrinc.com/24835/ (accessed Feb. 10, 2008).
2. Joint Commission Resources: Meeting the revised EM standards. *Environment of Care News* 10:7, Sep. 2007.

Chapter 2

Addressing Emergency Planning Issues

Catastrophic emergencies are a threat to any health care organization, regardless of size, scope, or location. A single emergency temporarily can affect demand for services, but multiple emergencies that occur at the same time or occur one after another can have serious consequences on patient safety and an organization's ability to provide care, treatment, and services for an extended length of time. This is particularly true in situations in which the community cannot adequately support the health care organization. Power failures, water and fuel shortages, flooding, and communications breakdowns are just a few of the hazards that can disrupt care and pose risks to staff and the organization as a whole. The disastrous and long-lasting effects of Hurricane Katrina in 2005 clearly demonstrated this fact.

Although no hospital or Medicare-/Medicaid-based long term care program can predict the nature of a future emergency or predict the date of its arrival, organizations can and should plan for managing the consequences of emergencies. Planning for emergencies precedes any management efforts, focusing on issues such as identifying events that could affect demand for services or the ability to provide those services and working with community partners to mitigate, prepare for, respond to, and recover from an incident that occurs in a health care organization or its community.

This chapter describes how health care organizations can address emergency planning issues necessary to establish a comprehensive Emergency Operations Plan (EOP). (*See* Chapter 3 for more information on the EOP.) Sidebar 2-1 (page 8) details the Joint Commission's expectations related to addressing emergency management planning issues.

Managing the Consequences of Emergencies

An emergency in a health care organization or in its community can suddenly and significantly affect demand for its services or its ability to provide those services. The standard focused on in this chapter describes the comprehensive planning and work necessary to establish an EOP that will allow for an effective response. The standard includes several elements found in the previous emergency management standards, such as the hazard vulnerability analysis (HVA). It also includes some new requirements, such as the need to establish an inventory of on-site assets and resources that would be needed during an emergency and to determine a way to monitor those assets and resources during an emergency, as described in the following sections.

Leadership Participation

More than any other aspect of environment of care (EC) management, the emergency management function might have the greatest potential for keeping organization leaders awake at night. Hurricanes and natural disasters, terrorist threats, and other emergencies are, by their nature, unpredictable and unplanned.

Effectively managing emergencies requires the commitment and collaboration of organization leaders to anticipate possible events and their effects, and to effectively respond and recover from them. Leaders, by their very definition as individuals who set expectations, develop plans, and implement procedures, must take responsibility for emergency management.

The importance of leadership to the emergency management process is spelled out in this standard, which requires organization leaders to actively participate in emergency management planning. In the hospital setting, leaders include those of the medical staff. In long term care organizations, the leaders involved in this process should include the administrator, the medical director, the nursing leader, and other clinical leaders.

Leaders who are involved in the emergency management process must promote staff participation because it is crucial

Sidebar 2-1.
Applicable Emergency Management Standard

The organization plans for managing the consequences of emergencies.

This standard requires the following:
- The organization's leaders (including those of the medical staff in hospitals and including the administrator, medical director, nursing leader, and other clinical leaders in long term care facilities) actively participate in emergency management planning.
- The organization conducts a hazard vulnerability analysis (HVA) to identify events that could affect demand for its services or its ability to provide those services, the likelihood of those events occurring, and the consequences of those events. The HVA is evaluated at least annually, as required by one of the elements of performance (EPs).
- The organization (together with its community partners in both hospitals and critical access hospitals) prioritizes those hazards, threats, and events identified in its HVA.
- When developing its Emergency Operations Plan, the organization communicates its needs and vulnerabilities to community emergency response agencies and identifies the capabilities of its community in meeting their needs.

For each emergency identified in its HVA, the organization defines the following:
- Mitigation activities designed to reduce the risk of and potential damage due to an emergency
- Preparedness activities that will organize and mobilize essential resources
- Response strategies and actions to be activated during the emergency
- Recovery strategies and actions designed to help restore the systems that are critical to resuming normal care, treatment, and services
- The organization keeps a documented inventory of the assets and resources it has on site that would be needed during an emergency. At a minimum, this would be personal protective equipment; water; fuel; and medical, surgical, and pharmaceutical staff, resources, and assets in a hospital or critical access hospital. Note: The inventory is evaluated at least annually as required in one EP.
- The organization establishes methods for monitoring quantities of assets and resources during an emergency.
- The objectives, scope, performance, and effectiveness of the organization's emergency management planning efforts are evaluated at least annually.

to a successful approach to this issue. For this reason, leaders must frequently communicate the importance of emergency management and encourage everyone in the organization to focus on emergency management as an ongoing concern. Emergency management must not be a one-time-only effort; the message about emergency management must continue over time. In addition to the requirements of the standard, this approach is supported by organizations such as the American College of Healthcare Executives, which calls on leaders to actively participate in emergency management planning by taking a number of steps, such as adopting an all-hazards planning framework that fits within overall community plans.[1]

To become involved, leaders should review the emergency management standards to make sure they understand the requirements. They can then examine the functions that are affected by the standards and look for ways to add or mix these requirements and ideas into existing processes to create a coordinated, organizationwide, and proactive approach to emergency management. Leaders need to participate in the emergency management planning process so that the organization can set priorities and leadership can allocate financial, information, physical, and human resources to support these priorities and associated processes. In addition, leaders can encourage communication and cooperation among all staff to implement emergency management processes.

> **Be Prepared Tip**
> **Involving Medical Staff Leaders**
> The planning process for emergency management should have direct involvement and input from organization leadership. Input from medical staff leadership is particularly important because the medical staff will play a critical role in response efforts.

Although leaders must drive the emergency management planning process and remain engaged in order to ensure that adequate resources are available, Joint Commission standards do not require the chief executive officer, administrator, or other leader to actually coordinate the ongoing emergency management processes after they have been established. Rather, the leadership involvement requirement emphasizes the need to coordinate these activities with accountability for inaction and for success resting with leadership.

> **Be Prepared Tip**
> **Involving the Entire Staff**
> As the planning effort begins to take form, include representatives from across departments. They in turn can get opinions from others in their respective departments. This method of getting feedback makes all employees a part of the process.

Conducting an HVA and Prioritizing

One of the first tasks involved in effective emergency management planning is conducting an HVA. An HVA identifies potential threats, risks, and emergencies and the potential impact these emergencies might have. The Joint Commission requires critical access hospitals, hospitals, and long term care organizations to conduct an HVA to identify events that could affect demand for services or the ability to provide those services, the likelihood of those events occurring, and the consequences of those events. For hospitals, this also includes a requirement that this process include collaboration with community partners. The organizations also need to prioritize those hazards, threats, and events identified in the HVA.

The all-hazards approach to emergency management is a comprehensive approach that enables organizations to be prepared to manage any number or type of emergencies. It facilitates mitigation, preparedness, response, and recovery based on the broad scope of what could happen within the organization and its community. The HVA is a formal assessment of the risks that can potentially affect the health care facility and cause the staff to implement the all-hazards emergency plan. The emergencies identified in the HVA must be prioritized in coordination with the community so that appropriate mitigation, preparedness, response, and recovery activities can be undertaken.

The HVA requirement is a familiar one to health care organizations, which even prior to Joint Commission requirements for an HVA, informally considered potential threats. For example, a hospital in Florida knows that it must address hurricanes but not blizzards. The opposite is true for a long term care organization in Minnesota. However, the standard calling for the management of the consequences of emergencies indicates that a more formal analysis process is necessary.

Organizations that fail to invest adequate time in the HVA process leave themselves vulnerable as emergency events are escalating. Planning for every possible emergency is not realistic, but organizations should assess as many threats as possible. For example, organizations during the past several years have had to come to terms with the need to "think the unthinkable." Before September 11, 2001, crashing a civilian airplane into a high-rise building was unthinkable. But it happened. Anthrax attacks in fall 2001 also made the possibility of biological, chemical, and radiological incidents more real. All health care organizations need to be prepared to face such disasters, requiring them to redefine the realm of possibility.

> **Be Prepared Tip**
> **An Evolving Hazards Vulnerability Analysis (HVA)**
> An HVA should not be a one-time event, but a continuous process that is thorough and that helps shape an organization's plans for emergency management and response.

An organization can perform an HVA in many ways; there is no right or wrong way. Any system that works effectively should be used and referenced in the EOP. Some systems use a quantitative scoring method to rank the potential emergencies, but this is not essential. The key is that each organization must identify the events to which it must be prepared to react. A description of one approach follows.

Be Prepared Tip

Develop a Hazard Vulnerability Analysis (HVA) Tool

An organization can develop its own HVA tool by classifying hazards and placing them on a simple grid format. Hazards can be ranked by using numbering such as 1 = could occur or high, 2 = might occur or moderate, and 3 = could never occur or no likelihood. The impact on the organization can be rated by using a high-, moderate-, low-, or no-impact ranking. Then the ranked hazards and impacts can be linked with the organization's resources that could be affected. Identifying how each resource will be affected by each hazard becomes the basis of how the organization will plan for an emergency and respond to it.

An HVA is based on an "all-hazards" approach. Thus, compiling a list of any possible hazards, emergencies, or incidents that the organization might experience is the place to start. When assembling this list, staff should be careful not to limit the list only to incidents that health care organizations have traditionally thought of as disasters, such as hurricanes, earthquakes, tornadoes, and other natural disasters. Internal events dealing with facility damage or system failures should also be considered, as should intentional man-made incidents, such as chemical and biological terrorism. Staff should remember to list mass-casualty events, such as transportation accidents, that might be commonly experienced. This list is best generated in a brainstorming session or something similar, during which every idea is written down without censorship or editorial comment. A review of community historical data might also provide additional list items.

When brainstorming about possible incidents, organizations often classify events in HVAs as being internal or external. An internal emergency involves the loss of a critical resource or resources needed to operate an organization. It is generally limited in scope to a specific facility, and, due to infrastructure damage, the facility might need to be evacuated. Examples appear in Table 2-1 (page 11). An external emergency is focused outside a facility. In some circumstances, an external emergency can also directly affect a facility's ability to keep operating. Examples of external emergencies appear in Table 2-2 (page 11).

After the brainstorming session, the organization should begin assessing the various items on the list. One place to start is with the *likelihood,* or *probability,* of occurrence. The local emergency planning committee in the community should be able to help with this. Very likely, data on the frequency of given incidents already exist. Your community might even have an HVA of its own that can provide a place to start, but it might not fully address all the health care organization's potential emergencies.

Disasters that have occurred before in the community and/or the organization will move toward the top of the list of issues to be addressed, whereas those with essentially no possibility of occurrence will migrate to the bottom. In between, staff will determine relative probability of occurrence. For example, earthquakes would be high on the list of potential emergencies for an organization in Southern California, but blizzards would be low on the list. Power failure and flood might be somewhere in between.

Probable impact is the next factor in the analysis. If the event occurs, staff should consider how it will affect the organization. Could lives be lost or the health and safety of individuals be threatened? If the answer to either of these questions is "yes," the hazard moves up on the list. If the answer is "no," staff should consider other ways in which the organization could be affected, such as disruption of services or damage to the facility, systems, or equipment. Damage affecting some services will be more important than others. Loss of use of an outpatient waiting area, for instance, would be far less critical than loss of a surgical suite in a hospital setting. Would an evacuation be necessary? Staff determine if the recovery would

Be Prepared Tip

Broadening the Definition of *Disaster*

Organizations should be careful not to limit the list of possible hazards, emergencies, or events to those they have traditionally thought of as *disasters*—hurricanes, earthquakes, tornadoes, and other natural disasters. Consider internal events dealing with facility damage or system failures and man-made events. And don't forget the more commonly occurring mass-casualty events, such as transportation accidents. Finally, consider that health care organizations are vulnerable to more local varieties of terrorism, perhaps carried out by a disgruntled employee or care recipient.

Table 2-1. Examples of What Could Lead to Internal Emergencies

Fire, smoke, or irritant fumes • Operating room • Recovery room • Emergency department • Intensive care units • Care recipient and nonpatient care areas Loss of environmental support services • Heat • Water supply • Air-conditioning • Sterilization • Electrical power • Telecommunications – Paging – Telephones • Computer networks	Loss of medical gases • Oxygen • Compressed air • Vacuum suction Explosion Police actions Acts of terrorism • Hostage situation • Workplace violence • Bioterrorism or nuclear terrorism • Hazardous materials release – Radiation – Toxic chemicals

Source: Joint Commission Resources: *Guide to Emergency Management Planning in Health Care.* Oakbrook Terrace, IL: Joint Commission on Accreditation of Healthcare Organizations, 2002.

Table 2-2. Examples of What Could Lead to External Emergencies

Hazardous weather • Earthquake • Hurricane • Flood • Tornado • Blizzard Regional power outage Civil disturbance Terrorism (including bioterrorism) Urban or wildland fires	Commercial transportation accidents • Train derailments • Air crashes • Multiple highway casualties • Hazardous materials release – Radiation – Toxic chemicals Evacuation of neighboring facilities • Ambulatory care organizations • Behavioral health care organizations • Hospitals • Long term care organizations

Source: Joint Commission Resources: *Guide to Emergency Management Planning in Health Care.* Oakbrook Terrace, IL: Joint Commission on Accreditation of Healthcare Organizations, 2002.

be relatively quick and simple or if it would be involved, costly, and long-lasting. Staff then adjust the ranking of the potential hazards according to the answers.

Another aspect of severity of impact is the community's perception of the health care organization. An organization's perception or image is extremely valuable to that organization. An organization's reputation can be damaged by its lack of preparedness to manage a foreseeable incident. This could also have legal ramifications. Failure to live up to community expectations could result in the loss of the community's trust, thus damaging the organization's reputation and potentially affecting its marketability and financial standing. Again, staff might adjust the ordering of list elements, as appropriate, to consider this possibility.

The long-term effect of an emergency also should be a consideration. For example, if an influx of contaminated patients should arrive at a facility, and the contaminant is contained, the loss of life would probably be minimal and the short-term effects relatively minor; however, to address contamination issues, a hospital might have to take the emergency department off-line for some period of time. The long-term effects of this aspect of the emergency could be very significant, and thus this type of emergency could be moved up on the priority list. The final factors that merit consideration are the organization's own preparedness

BE PREPARED TIP

Understanding Community Roles

In a communitywide emergency, all responders and all health care organizations are interdependent. For this reason, it is important that all responding agencies understand what services each can provide and what support each will need from other sources. In other words, it is essential that the health care organization understands how it is supporting the community and conversely how the community is supporting the organization.

status and the community's level of preparedness. If one of the high-ranking incidents on the list took place tomorrow, how well would the organization manage the incident? Would other organizations in the community be able to provide assistance? If the organization is not prepared to handle the incident, it should focus more attention on preparing for that potential hazard than it would for the hazards covered by well-established plans. A gap analysis helps to identify incidents for which the organization is not prepared and the steps that it can take to rectify the situation. If community resources could not be called on for assistance in addressing the incident, staff should move the incident up on the list. This analysis might result in some less-probable events being moved up on the list due to the fact that the most anticipated events are usually those for which the organization and community are already most prepared.

Reviewing the HVA with other emergency response agencies in the community ensures other compatibilities. Again, although there will undoubtedly be differences based on the different concerns of various agencies, there should be similarities in the areas of natural disasters and weather emergencies.

BE PREPARED TIP

Involve Patients and the Community in Planning

The elderly, children, and people with disabilities—whose lives depend on the strength of emergency planning—must be involved in the emergency planning process. Forming partnerships with regional agencies and organizations that serve as advocates for children, the elderly, and those with special needs can be beneficial in both assessing needs and educating these populations about emergency and disaster planning.

As part of developing the HVA, integration with local and regional emergency management agencies is critical. The standard under discussion recognizes that emergency planning should not be done in a vacuum. Hospitals and critical access hospitals should review their planning process to encourage community cooperation in planning for emergency management, to integrate the resources of the health care organization with those in the community, and to make sure everyone agrees on levels of responsibility.

Health care organizations must understand how they support the community and how the community can support them in an emergency. This requires the participation of health care organizations in community planning activities that extend beyond participation with the immediate community. These activities might include involvement with the local emergency planning committee or perhaps the state emergency management organization. Some communities have had the opportunity to participate in emergency management training sponsored by the Department of Homeland Security. Participation in this type of event is an asset that should be highlighted in the plan.

The completed list of potential hazards will now have those events that merit the most attention near the top, whether because of probability of occurrence, impact on the organization, or level of preparedness. Those less serious and not as likely to happen should be near the bottom. Although the ranking is dependent on subjective judgment and evaluation of the various considerations discussed previously, there should be some rationale for general placement on the list, although it might be difficult to distinguish the placement of two events that are sequenced consecutively. Two organizations within the same community will probably have differing analyses, but an earthquake should not be at the top of one list and the bottom of another.

Organizations might also wish to ask their legal counsel to review the HVAs to address the organizations' acceptance of risk as implied in the HVAs. Staff should also include the HVA in their annual evaluation of the EC management plan in terms of objectives, scope, performance, and effectiveness. Sidebar 2-2 (page 13) provides information about how to identify the limitations of hazard lists used as part of the HVA process, whereas Sidebar 2-3 (page 14) offers ideas about how to ensure that an HVA identifies realistic threats to the organization.

BE PREPARED TIP

Fostering Ongoing Community Connections

In the midst of an emergency is not the best time to introduce yourself to community leaders. Organization leadership should have a relationship with other community responders before an emergency occurs. This relationship should be fostered, and open communication should occur between all community response entities. If such communication does not occur, serious consequences can result from assumptions that might be inaccurate. To build a relationship with community leaders, organizations can hold periodic meetings with police and fire officials, public health officials, and leadership from other organizations in the community, such as schools, corporations, and universities. This will ensure that roles and responsibilities are clearly defined and that expectations match what actually can be provided by each stakeholder.

Sidebar 2-2.

Recognizing Problems Inherent in Hazard Lists

Hazard lists pose two problems. The first problem is the possibility of exclusion or omission: There is always a potential for new and unexpected hazards, which is part of why maintaining an all-hazards capability is important.

The second problem is that such lists involve groupings, which can affect subsequent analysis. A list might give the impression that hazards are independent of one another, when in fact they are often related (for example, an earthquake might give rise to dam failure). Lists might group under one category very different causes or sequences of events that require different types of response. For example, "flood" might include dam failure, cloudbursts, or heavy rain upstream. Lists also might group a whole range of consequences under the category of a single hazard. "Terrorism," for example, could include use of conventional explosives against people or critical infrastructure; nuclear detonation; release of lethal chemical, biological, or radiological material; and more. "Hurricane" might include not only high winds, storm surge, and battering waves, but even the weakened, post-landfall tropical storm system that can cause inland flooding. It might be necessary, as the hazard analysis evolves, to refine the list of hazards.

Source: Excerpted from Federal Emergency Management Agency: *State and Local Guide (SLG) 101: Guide for All-Hazard Emergency Operations Planning.* 1996. http://www.fema.gov/plan/gaheop.shtm (accessed Oct. 2, 2007).

Communicating with the Community About Needs

The standard requiring the management of an emergency's consequences requires a health care organization to communicate with its community about the organization's needs and how the community can help meet those needs. The previous standards required health care organizations to establish with their communities the organization's role in an emergency. But in some cases, as for example with a long term care organization, the organization might not have a specific role in an emergency. The organization would still have to have its needs met, though, and the organization might have to rely on the community to meet those needs. Consequently, the organization has an obligation to communicate its needs and understand if and how the community will be able assist in meeting those needs.

Involving and communicating with the community about emergency preparedness is critical to an effective response and recognizes the fact that organizations cannot develop an emergency management program in isolation. By collaborating with the community in the planning process, an organization can develop stronger relationships with other community partners that promote greater understanding of the interactions that will be crucial during any type of disaster.

Organizations seeking to meet this requirement can think about existing relationships that might already be in place with the community. For example, most hospitals and long term care organizations have relationships and agreements in place with the public health department, emergency medical services, fire department, and police department. Hospitals are

What Are the Risks?

As part of a 2006 survey, emergency preparedness officials were asked whether their hospitals were at risk for any particular hazards or threats. Although the most common concern was hazardous materials, weather-related disasters also ranked high on the list.

Human-made hazards:

- Hazardous materials: 76.0%
- Terrorism: 47.1%
- Nuclear: 25.9%
- Military installation: 17.9%

Natural hazards:

- Winter storms: 67.3%
- Tornado: 62.1%
- Floods: 41.9%
- Extreme heat: 33.0%
- Earthquake: 24.7%
- Hurricane: 24.5%
- Wildfire: 16.7%
- Dams: 12.4%
- Landslide: 4.5%
- Tsunami: 2.4%
- Volcano: 1.4%

Source: Braun B., et al.: Integrating hospitals into community emergency preparedness planning. *Ann Intern Med* 144:799–811, Jun. 2006.

Sidebar 2-3.

Getting Input

A hazard vulnerability analysis (HVA) is effective only if it identifies realistic threats to the organization. Ensuring that all potential events are identified requires input from multidisciplinary groups. Some organizations choose to involve the entire emergency management committee in the HVA process. The committee identifies and prioritizes risks related to security, facility, safety, infection control, and radiation issues. When assessing the risks in each area, it is important to have the appropriate people make the evaluation. For example, the facility manager should evaluate facility issues. This person is very aware of the potential risks to which his or her facility might be subjected and what systems would be most affected by a particular emergency. Consider this example: An organization was updating its HVA, and the emergency management committee assumed that an electrical power outage would be a catastrophic issue for the facility. However, the facility manager pointed out that due to backup power systems, a power outage would not be catastrophic, but a water outage could shut down the entire institution in a short period of time. His input into the HVA process helped redirect the organization's focus and shape its response efforts.

Organizations should also include senior leadership in the HVA process. Organization leaders should be aware of what the emergency management committee considers potential threats to the institution, given that leadership is ultimately responsible for making critical decisions during a crisis.

also likely to have relationships with city and county officials, local doctors, public schools, utility providers, the media, and other important components of the community. Hospitals and long term care organizations should also work with the community's emergency preparedness planning group. Communicating about organization needs and vulnerabilities and the ability of the community to meet those organization needs is a natural extension of this effort.

Mitigation, Preparedness, Response, and Recovery

For each emergency identified in the HVA, organizations must then address the four phases of emergency management activities: mitigation, preparedness, response, and recovery.

Mitigation activities are designed to reduce the risk of and potential damage due to an emergency. These activities may be part of other efforts to meet codes and standards. For example, compliance with the National Fire Protection Association's *Life Safety Code*® (NFPA 101®)* is designed to reduce the impact of a fire in a health care facility. Or, the presence of an emergency electrical generator mitigates the risk of an electrical power failure.

Mitigation begins with identifying hazards that could affect the organization and analyzing the vulnerability to those hazards of care recipients, personnel, facilities, telecommunications, and informational resources. Conducting an HVA is generally one of the first mitigation activities that an organization undertakes.

Some experts categorize mitigation activities as hard or soft.[2] *Hard* mitigation activities "harden" a facility to make it withstand a disaster with little active human intervention. This traditional strategy involves constructing the built environment to withstand natural hazards, such as adding uninterruptible power supplies, standby power generators, fire suppression systems, and structures that can withstand damages from wind and earthquakes. *Soft* mitigation activities reduce the effect of disasters that cannot be adequately alleviated by hard mitigation measures. Such activities might include sandbagging against a flood.[2]

Decisions regarding which mitigation activities to pursue should be made based on a cost-benefit analysis, weighing the costs of both the losses and the needed action for mitigation against the likelihood of the disaster. Some mitigation activities cost next to nothing, such as placing certain flammable materials in fireproof containers; others require significant investment, such as battery-powered lighting for all floors and added structural modifications to protect against collapse during floods or hurricanes.

Preparedness refers to activities that will organize and mobilize essential resources. Preparedness involves planning how to respond if a disaster occurs. This step has been the foundation of health care emergency planning for many years. Some important preparedness steps include the following:

- Creating an inventory of resources that might be needed in an emergency, including prearranged agreements with vendors and health care networks
- Maintaining an ongoing planning process
- Holding staff orientation on basic response actions
- Implementing organizationwide exercises to test the plan

A checklist that could be used as a starting point for backup resources and supplies that might be needed appears in Table 2-3 (page 16).

Response includes the strategies and actions that are activated during an emergency. It involves treating victims, reducing secondary impact to the organization, and controlling the negative effects of emergency situations. How an organization responds to an emergency is absolutely critical. As with preparedness, many health care facilities, particularly hospitals, might be well equipped to manage this phase because treating victims is what they do on a daily basis. Other health care organizations might not be as well equipped to treat victims (for example, when a long term care organization receives trauma and burn victims from a terrorist attack in the community, or when a sudden influx of patients occurs in a hospital in the middle of the night when sufficient staff are not available). Response activities are best divided into actions that all staff must take when confronted by an emergency, such as implementing "RACE" in response to a fire (**R**emoval of patients from danger, **A**larm activation, **C**losing of doors, and **E**vacuating of staff), and those taken by management, such as initiating the plan, assessing the situation, issuing warning and notification announcements, setting objectives and priorities, and serving as a liaison with external groups.

The *recovery* phase involves restoring the systems that are critical to resuming normal care, treatment, and services. In other words, how will the organization get back to business? The plan, of course, depends on the nature of the incident, whether the emergency is ongoing, whether the facility itself is affected, and whether the local area or region is still affected. The recovery phase of the EOP should specify recovery steps or stages, similar to how implementation of the emergency management plan is described in stages or steps. Financial, staffing, and service implications need to be considered.

Recovery planning also includes such things as insurance coverage and inventory records. In addition, the facility must consider management authorizations for purchasing, document security, and outsourcing of services that temporarily cannot be provided internally. The plan should also include readjusting staff schedules during stand-down, if necessary. Employees who leave the facility might not be able to return immediately to their regular work schedules if they have to attend to their families and homes. Getting back to providing care is integral to disaster recovery under some circumstances, and this will incorporate the concerns of affected staff members and physician offices. Repair of facilities might also be an issue. Mental health issues of staff, as described in Chapter 7, should be con-

* *Life Safety Code*® is a registered trademark of the National Fire Protection Association, Quincy, MA.

Table 2-3. Backup Supplies Checklist

Organizations should consider the following as a starting point in their process of identifying backup supplies that might be needed in emergencies. Organizations must be prepared to function completely on their own for at least 24 to 48 hours, in the case of an emergency in which federal resources would be mobilized, and preferably for up to 72 to 96 hours.

Basic materials:

- Food
- Water
- Linens
- Blankets
- Flashlights
- Batteries
- Extension cords
- Stockpile rope
- Water-purifying tablets
- Flares
- Duct tape
- Markers
- Work gloves
- Brooms
- Masks
- Matches
- Sandbagging equipment
- Plywood (for windows)
- Physical map of the facility
- Utility system blueprints
- Fuel for generators
- Binoculars
- Victim tags
- Updated physical plan of facility and blueprints of utility systems

Basic tools:

- For fixing plumbing leaks
- For splicing cables
- For repairing or insulating electrical wiring

Backup communication devices:

- Walkie-talkies
- Radios
- Cellular telephones
- Other devices that would function if utility systems failed

Spare parts:

- Full list should be developed of critical equipment parts.

Medical supplies:

- Full list should be developed, including supplies that can be expected for use in treating certain types of injuries, such as multiple fractures, serious cuts, or electrocutions. These can be predicted for almost all disasters.
- Portable lifesaving equipment such as manual ventilators and gas systems
- Tape, gauze, needle assortments, endotracheal tubes, portable oxygen, defibrillators, splints, gloves, disinfectants

Pharmaceutical supplies:

- Full list should be developed based on what can be expected for use in treating care recipients and staff.
- Backup suppliers?
- Standing orders created?
- Credit lines preestablished?
- Phone number list placed with disasters supplies and at the command center?

Placement of backup/disaster supplies:

- In a nearby location outside the facility

Source: ECRI Institute. Plymouth Meeting, PA. May 2002. www.ecri.org (accessed Feb. 1, 2008). Reprinted with permission.

sidered. Even critiques of the disaster incident are part of the recovery process.

Assets and Resources

The revised standard addressing the management of the consequences of emergencies also includes new requirements for health care organizations related to assets and resources. One of the requirements under the standard is for the organization to keep a documented inventory of the assets and resources it has on site that would be needed during an emergency. The minimum inventory requirements include personal protective equipment; water; fuel; and staffing, medical, and pharmaceuticals resources and assets. For hospitals and critical access hospitals, surgical resources and assets are added to that minimum list. As part of another requirement, which is discussed later in this chapter, the inventory must be evaluated annually. The standard also requires organizations to establish a method for monitoring consumption of assets and resources during an emergency.

These new requirements tie in with the standard that is the focus of Chapter 5, requiring the management of resources and assets during emergencies. Organizations, however, cannot meet this requirement or effectively create an emergency management plan without first knowing exactly what they have. By keeping a documented inventory of these essential supplies, organizations can assess how emergencies identified in the HVA would impact the inventory. Organizations must keep track of assets and resources used during an emergency so that resources can be resupplied or, if not possible, rationed until recovery is possible. Monitoring resources and assets during an emergency also will provide for more effective emergency management by the organization in the future by providing a better understanding of what items are necessary.

Evaluating Planning Efforts

The final element of performance for the standard discussed in this chapter requires organizations to evaluate the objectives, scope, performance, and effectiveness of emergency management planning efforts at least annually. This requirement, which has been relocated from previous EC standards, is a precursor to developing and maintaining an EOP as required by the standard discussed in this chapter, and the standard calling for regular testing of an organization's EOP (*see* Chapter 10).

Evaluating the planning efforts' objectives means determining how well the planning effort accomplished what it set out to do. If the objectives are appropriately laid out at the beginning of the year, their assessment at the time of the evaluation can be very straightforward. The same objectives can be carried forward from year to year in the planning process if they remain appropriate.

The scope of the emergency management planning effort is defined by its breadth. Some planning efforts cover only one facility; others cover all facilities within a larger organization. Thus site information is part of the scope. For this portion of the annual evaluation, the organization assesses whether the planning effort's definition of scope remains appropriate or whether something has changed in the composition of the organization.

Emergency planning lacks meaning without performance measurement—a way to measure whether and how well the organization is planning and implementing its EOP. The performance-monitoring data that are collected for the EOP form the backbone of the performance section of the annual evaluation. Thus, it is appropriate that these data be presented, trended, and analyzed. Following an actual emergency, an organization collects and analyzes data related to its implementation of the EOP. In the absence of an actual emergency, data related to planned exercises and other items, such as effectiveness of training, should be collected and analyzed. Documentation provided by drill observers can provide relevant performance data on the adequacy of staff training, risks and needs, missing steps, and opportunities for improvement. A sample run chart that tracks the effectiveness of emergency management training appears in Figure 2-1 (page 18). Or, for example, performance measures might examine management and staff activity. By focusing on improving rather than on just getting by, organizations can choose a new aspect of performance to measure after effectiveness is demonstrated and return to monitor previous performance measures from time to time.

The section of the annual evaluation on the effectiveness of the emergency management planning process is subjective. This is where the responsible parties consider what went well during the previous year and what needs to be improved. It should also identify and lay out issues on the horizon and objectives for the coming year. The evaluation of the emergency management planning effort is a key troubleshooting activity. Being prepared means realizing what could go wrong before it does. No one can predict or address all possible contingencies, but several areas are often neglected during an initial response plan analysis. By considering the priority of potential emergencies, an organization can generate first-line and backup processes that convey critical information and are still flexible enough to address a wild card, such as a tight-fitting or torn decontamination suit.

One way to evaluate emergency management planning efforts is to bring an interdisciplinary and interdepartmental committee to the table. An interdepartmental and interdisciplinary team will likely identify the greatest number of issues to address in the plan.

Asking questions helps to identify weaknesses in planning efforts. However, exercises are the best way to discover problems with the plan and to identify areas that still need improvement. (*See* Chapter 10.)

The disaster readiness checklist published by the American Hospital Association following the September 11, 2001, attacks provides an overview of emergency management plans that should be reviewed by every health care organization. This appears as Table 2-4, page 19.

Figure 2-1. Sample Run Chart: Effectiveness of Emergency Management Training

This run chart shows that staff members demonstrate the highest level of understanding of the emergency management program one month after training occurs.

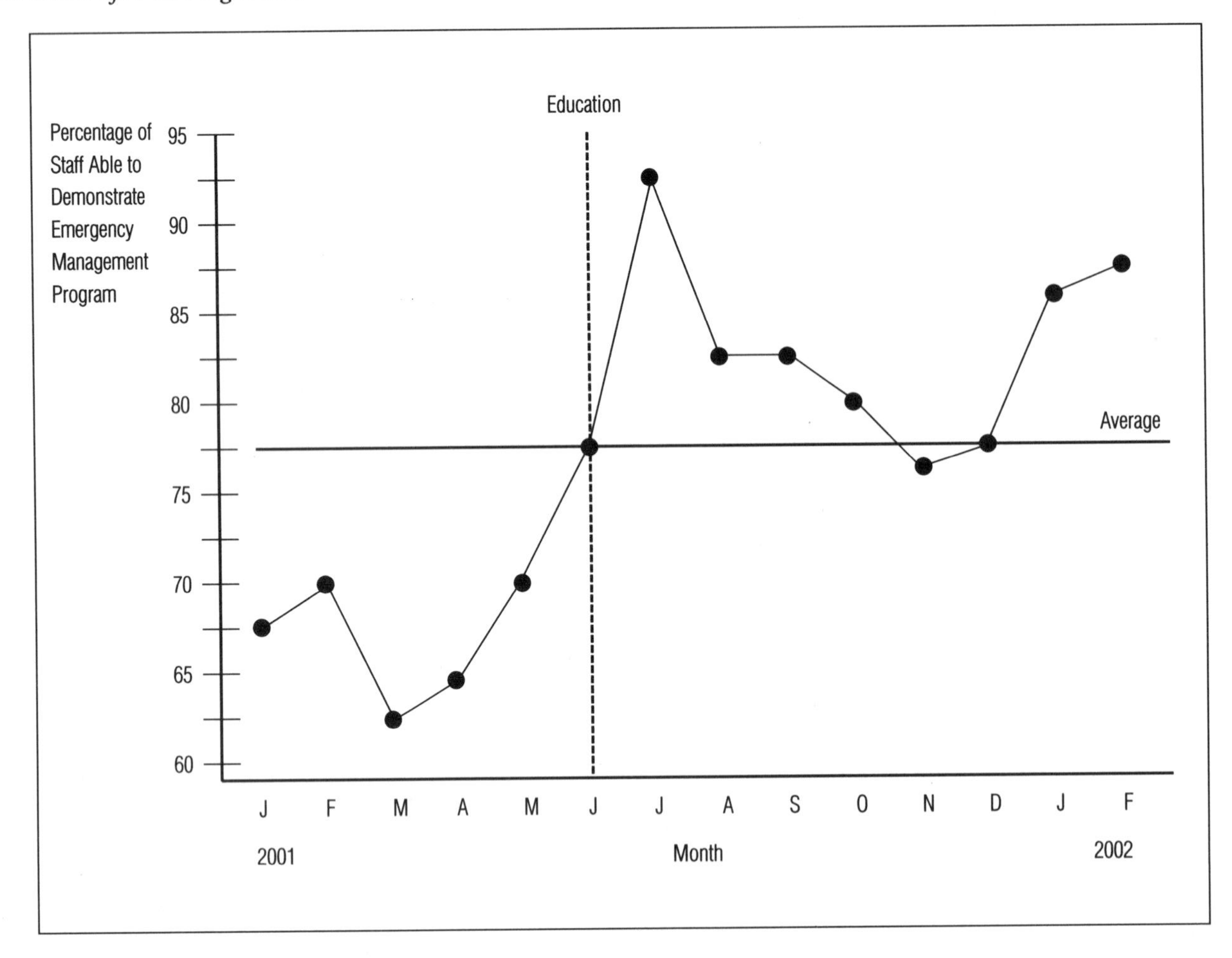

Source: Joint Commission Resources: *Performance Improvement in the Environment of Care.* Oakbrook Terrace, IL: Joint Commission on Accreditation of Healthcare Organizations, 2001.

Table 2-4. Disaster Readiness Checklist

- ❑ Focus your efforts on a general "all-hazards" plan that provides an adaptable framework for crisis situations. The terrorist attacks have revealed that the unimaginable can become reality.
- ❑ Upgrade your disaster plan. The attacks have dramatically altered the potential range of disasters communities might face. Be sure that your plan includes components for mass-casualty terrorism, including the potential for chemical or biological incidents.
- ❑ Connect with your community's emergency response agencies. This is a good time to integrate your plan with your community's rescue squad and police and fire departments. Specifically, make sure you have the latest contact numbers for key agencies and that they, in turn, have an up-to-date list of your organization's key contacts.
- ❑ Develop a plan to support the families of staff members. Staff members want and need assurances that their families are protected and cared for, especially if the incident involves chemical or biological exposure. This is likely to involve agencies and resources from the broader community.
- ❑ Develop a simplified patient registration procedure in the event of a very large number of casualties.
- ❑ Review your backup communications capabilities. Traditional telecommunications mechanisms can become overwhelmed. Pay special attention to backup communications mechanisms, such as Internet-based communication tools and even couriers.
- ❑ Ensure that essential information systems and data storage have off-site storage and recovery capabilities. In the event of a large-scale incident, you might have to rely on resources outside your own community.
- ❑ Be prepared to talk with your community and its leaders, lawmakers, and others about how your organization would deal with a mass-casualty event, especially an incident with large numbers of survivors. Also be prepared to provide a medical advisory to the mayor and other public officials who might be the primary foci of the media.
- ❑ Review your supply and inventory strategy. Many organizations have moved to "just in time" supply schedules, which keep enough supplies on hand to care for expected patients. Although state and federal resources will become available, communities might be "on their own" for at least 24 to 48 hours. Include the possibility that traditional transportation systems could be disabled.
- ❑ Examine how to protect the physical security of your organization by limiting access to the facility.
- ❑ If your organization is part of the National Disaster Medical System, review who the contact is within your organization and who the federal coordinator is in your area. If located in an urban area, determine if there is a Metropolitan Medical Response System plan in your community and know how it can complement the organization's own plan.
- ❑ Ensure that the organization and its medical staff report unexpected illness patterns to the public health department and, if appropriate, the Centers for Disease Control and Prevention.
- ❑ Finally, with the armed services calling up reserves (and individual states' National Guards) and the possibility that the Department of Health and Human Services' Office of Emergency Preparedness might need to call up response teams (Disaster Medical Assistance Team [DMAT], Disaster Mortuary Operational Response Team [DMORT], and Metropolitan Medical Response System [MMRS]), take time to inventory who on your staff, including medical staff, could get called, what your policies are for job retention and benefit continuation, and how activation might affect your operations.

Source: American Hospital Association. *Disaster Readiness Advisory #1: Disaster Readiness.* http://www.aha.orgaha/advisory/2001/01921-disaster-adv.html (accessed Mar. 10, 2008).

Sidebar 2-4.

Involving the Right People

Emergency management planning and implementation must be a team process and must involve key individuals within and outside the organization, including volunteers, agencies, and community contacts.

The Organization's Team

Emergency management planning should be a team process within the organization. A team approach brings increased creativity, knowledge, and experience to each phase of the emergency management planning process, including mitigation, preparedness, response, and recovery activities. A team provides a powerful and successful way to effect plan implementation. The team approach starts with a leader who is motivated to make emergency management work. This leader can be the safety officer or someone else. He or she should begin with the leadership from the organization's administration and the medical staff.

The goal in successful planning is to involve all the organization's facilities and departments, as they will all be affected and play a role in the emergency response. Representatives of many areas should be included, such as administration, risk management, safety and security, public relations, materials management, pharmacy, and clinical staff. Those individuals in charge of the organization's information management and patient safety departments also should be included.

Clinical staff, such as pharmacists, physicians, and nurses, have much to contribute in preparing for an emergency response. They will be providing care to disaster victims and can provide expertise during the planning process. For example, pharmacists develop formularies of medications for use at the disaster site and consider the ease of use, storage requirements, and shipping ability of the medications that will be dispensed and other formulary requirements such as the availability of potable water and security needs.[1] One of the key tasks of the emergency management planning team is to determine the most appropriate and effective incident command structure for the organization, as described in Chapter 3.

Emergency management planning teams might also include representatives from outside the organization. For example, the team might include representatives from the local emergency preparedness office; representatives from state health care organizations; a media representative (who can serve an important communication function during external natural disasters); a Red Cross representative; police officers; and representatives from fire, gas, electrical, and other utility companies.

Another key task of the emergency management planning team is to facilitate the creation of emergency response teams within the organization. Some organizations begin with the departments that are organization-based and active 24 hours per day, as appropriate. If the facility has several buildings, departments in the main building of the campus are the first to be considered. The planning team identifies representatives from these departments and brings them together with an experienced facilitator and a leader. This core group will establish basic ground rules and set the group's goals. Representatives should seek out opinions from others in their departments and be sure to involve the safety committee when it is appropriate. Most safety committees are already organized to address preparedness plans for both internal and external emergencies. A subcommittee reporting to the safety committee often performs the emergency management planning function.

Reference

1. Ames T.W., Montello M.J.: Management consultation: Role of pharmacists on disaster response teams. *Am J Health Syst Pharm* 56:716–718, Apr. 15, 1999.

Sidebar 2-5.

Selected Emergency Management Planning Questions

- What credible threats might the organization need to respond to?
- Who needs to be involved in this response, both inside and outside the organization?
- What response services must the organization provide?
- What provisions need to be made to provide services to specific populations currently served by the organization and those in the community?
- What is the "big-picture" response system in the community and nation, and where does the organization fit in?
- Is the organization's emergency management plan both compatible with and complementary to plans developed by other health care organizations in the community?
- Who is in charge of the organization's response, and what aspects do these people handle? What role does each key responder play?
- In addition to casualty care, what are the other elements of preparation for the organization?
- What staff will be needed to handle an emergency? How will the organization ensure the availability of those staff? What are the contingency plans if staff cannot get to work or, as might be the case in an incident or a threat involving biological agents, don't wish to report to work because of concern about their own safety?
- How will the organization handle "contaminated" casualties?
- How will the organization practice its response to emergencies and assess its performance?
- How do leaders assess the organization's state of readiness?
- Where do leaders currently go and where should they go to get reliable, accurate, and accepted information about emergency response?

Source: Joint Commission Resources: *Guide to Emergency Management Planning Health Care.* Oakbrook Terrace, IL: Joint Commission on Accreditation of Healthcare Organizations, 2002.

Sidebar 2-6.

Nursing Homes and Public Health Emergencies

To date, most health care preparedness planning efforts are focused on hospital and first responder preparedness. Nevertheless, we know that the elderly population is particularly vulnerable to bioterrorism and other public health emergencies due to their complex physical, medical, and psychosocial needs. The potential role and question of preparedness on the part of nursing homes has emerged in local and national preparedness discussions. However, we have little understanding of the extent to which nursing homes have planned for and/or have been incorporated into local or regional planning efforts.

A recent Agency for Healthcare Research and Quality study of planning activities among nursing homes in five states concludes that nursing homes have prepared for natural disasters but have given very little thought to bioterrorism. Facilities reported having disaster plans in place, some more comprehensive than others, and reviewing these plans with nursing staff at orientation and during regular in-service training. Disaster plans appeared to focus on the natural disasters most prevalent in a region (for example, wild fires, earthquakes, floods, hurricanes). Only a few facilities reported including policies and procedures specific to bioterrorism in their disaster plans.

The report noted concerns about caring for special patient populations that require specialized equipment or nursing care during an emergency. In particular, participants were concerned about patients with Alzheimer's and other cognitive impairments. Many facilities caring for these patients have locked facilities with high-tech monitoring systems that could easily fail during power loss. Participants also were concerned about the logistical difficulties involved in moving or evacuating patients with limited physical abilities. Linked to concerns about patient care were concerns about staffing. Participants were concerned about maintaining staffing levels because nursing staff would undoubtedly want to care for their own families or might have difficulty getting to work.

(continued)

Sidebar 2-6, *continued*

Nursing Homes and Public Health Emergencies

Several issues raised could be of concern to the larger health care community. These include the following:

- Maintaining adequate pharmaceutical and medical supplies
- The ability of generators to support an entire facility and the adequacy of fuel supplies
- Feeding the resident population and keeping them adequately hydrated

The results also suggest a number of potential roles nursing homes could play in the event of a public health emergency. Nearly all participants reported they could accept transferred residents back from area hospitals to free up bed space in those facilities. Most facilities acknowledged the possibility of receiving additional patients from the community and were willing to accommodate those patients if they could. In doing so, however, they had two major concerns: patient acuity and staffing. Many facilities specialize in caring for patients with certain conditions. Thus, one facility might be able to take a transferred ventilator patient whereas another could not. This suggests that area hospitals wanting to transfer patients need to know what the nursing homes in their area are skilled in. Nursing homes also need staff with the knowledge and expertise in providing care to higher acuity patients if they accept them.

Nursing homes could provide a variety of additional resources during an emergency, including basic medical care and short-term shelter. Participants agreed that nursing staff had the skills to provide a certain level of medical care to outside community members. They suggested staff could provide vaccinations, basic first aid, or triage services.

Source: Adapted from Root E.D., Amozegar J.B., Bernard S.: *Nursing Homes in Public Health Emergencies: Special Needs and Potential Roles.* Agency for Healthcare Research and Quality, AHRQ pub. no. 07-0029-1, May 2007. http://www.ahrq.gov/prep/nursinghomes/report.htm (accessed Oct. 2, 2007).

Coordinating with the Media

The media can provide health care organizations and the communities in which they operate with a powerful means of communicating during disasters. This has far-reaching consequences for organizations experiencing the effects of an emergency.

Considering the role of the media should play a part in emergency planning efforts because emergency management responses are improved when the media are given accurate and current information. In a large, regional emergency, the media might be one of the only available communication routes. Organizations might wish to consider how to engage in integrated communication planning, coordination, and public education as part of the emergency management planning process. One place to start is to discuss the issue with other community stakeholders and organizations involved in emergency response planning to review and adapt communications.

Finally, it should be noted that the media's sources also might be unavailable, so organizations work with local and/or regional emergency operations command systems to be a part of their linked communication networks.

Strategies for delivering information to the public and employees through the media are discussed in greater detail in Chapters 3 and 4.

Table 2-5. A Comprehensive Approach to Planning for Managing the Consequences of Emergencies*

To define a comprehensive approach to identifying risks and mobilizing an effective response within the organization as well as in collaboration and coordination with essential response partners in the community, the following four elements must be in place:

1. Leaders, including those of the medial staff, actively participate in emergency planning.
2. A hazard vulnerability analysis (HVA)† is conducted to identify events that could affect demand for services or the ability to provide services, the likelihood of those events occurring, and the consequences of those events.
3. The establishment, in coordination with community partners, of priorities among the potential hazards, threats, and events identified in the HVA.
4. Communication of organization needs and vulnerabilities to community emergency response agencies and identification of the capabilities of the community in meeting needs.
5. For each emergency identified in its HVA, the organization defines the following:
   - Mitigation activities to reduce the risk of and potential damage due to an emergency
   - Preparedness activities that will organize and mobilize essential resources
   - Response strategies and actions to be activated during the emergency
   - Recovery strategies and actions designed to help restore the systems that are critical to resuming normal care, treatment, and services
6. The organization keeps a documented inventory of assets and resources it has on site that would be needed during an emergency (at a minimum, personal protective equipment; water; fuel; and staffing, medical, and pharmaceuticals resources and assets for long term care organizations; critical access hospitals and hospitals also must add surgical resources to that minimum list.
7. A method is established for monitoring quantities of assets and resources during an emergency.

* This list is required for Joint Commission–accredited critical access hospitals, hospitals, and long term care organizations.

† HVA (hazard vulnerability analysis): The identification of potential emergencies and the direct and indirect effects these emergencies may have on the health care organization's operations and the demand for its services.

Case Example: A Coordinated Emergency Response

Although the revised emergency management standards went into effect January 1, 2008, some organizations were actually already meeting the intent of these standards due to their exemplary emergency response efforts. The following example describes the emergency response of one health care system to one of the largest natural disasters in our nation's history.

At the end of August 2005, Hurricane Katrina struck Louisiana, Alabama, and Mississippi, leaving behind devastation, destruction, and thousands of people in desperate need of health care with nowhere to go. Baptist Health System, a five-hospital system located in San Antonio, Texas, received some of these displaced patients and effectively met their health care needs while continuing to serve its own patients and community.

Shortly after the hurricane hit, the governor of Louisiana and the governors of surrounding states, including Texas, began talking about evacuating people from Louisiana. The governor of Texas agreed to house evacuees and began coordinating through the state emergency management (EM) agency where people needing health care would go.

"Our organization participates in a regional emergency planning group called Regional Medical Operations Center (RMOC), along with representatives from other hospitals throughout the area, subject matter experts—such as epidemiologists and radiation experts—the public health department, and EM services. The RMOC reports to and receives orders from San Antonio's Emergency Operations Center. The RMOC was notified about 10 hours before the evacuees began arriving that our area would be receiving patients," says Bill Waechter, director of emergency services and emergency management, Baptist Health System. "Due to the nature of the evacuation, we didn't know much more about the patients other than they were coming via airplane and approximately what time they would be landing."

Preparing for the Influx

After getting the news that they would be receiving patients, the five Baptist Health System Hospitals declared a standby Code Gray—the organization's disaster code—and began preparing for the influx of patients. The hospitals participated in a systemwide conference call, in which they discussed their disaster plans and how they were going to apply to this situation. "We talked about staffing, resources, communication, and other topics. As a group, we decided to establish alternate emergency areas within each of our facilities so as not to overtax our existing emergency departments (EDs) with the influx of Katrina evacuees. We were starting a holiday weekend (Labor Day), and we knew our EDs were going to be busy, regardless of the Katrina evacuees," says Waechter.

In addition to designating the alternate EDs, the hospitals pulled together multidisciplinary groups to staff these areas. A group included a hospitalist, nurses, a laboratory technician, an x-ray technician, and a representative from the registration department. This group was in charge of triaging the evacuees and facilitating their transfer into the facility.

When the plane carrying the evacuees landed, local EMS personnel met the plane, performed initial triage, and communicated with the RMOC about each patient. Based on bed availability and capacity within each of the hospitals participating in the RMOC, patients were distributed across the area.

(continued)

Case Example: A Coordinated Emergency Response, *continued*

Ensuring Effective Communication

Baptist Health System used various means of communication to ensure that all staff members were informed about the emergency and the status of the response. Baptist has an electronic Web-based communication tool that allows anyone across the system who has access to quickly see bed availability, resources, task force assignments, weather, and so forth. Multiple people throughout the system are in charge of maintaining different aspects of the tool to ensure that communication is up-to-the-minute and accurate. This tool also houses a chat room where significant events can be discussed and addressed. "During this particular emergency, we used the tool to communicate about resource needs. For example, one of the hospitals in the system needed wheelchairs and newborn isolettes. The hospital posted the need on the Web, and another hospital was able to provide the resources," says Waechter. To ensure that this system could keep operating during the emergency, the organization has a wireless local area network (LAN) that can serve as a backup. This LAN is independent of the organization's normal information technology structure. In addition to the Web communication tool, the organization also used 800 MHz ham radios to help facilitate communication.

Baptist Health System also addressed other issues during the emergency. For example, it controlled access to its facilities to ensure security, and it frequently monitored supply levels to ensure the appropriate amount of resources and supplies.

Receiving a sudden influx of patients from another state due to a hurricane does not happen every day. However, by having a well-considered, collaborative, and detailed emergency response program, the Baptist Health System hospitals were able to successfully treat Katrina victims and address their health and safety needs.

Source: Joint Commission Resources: Meeting the revised EM standards. *Environment of Care News* 10:9, Sep. 2007.

For Additional Assistance

In identifying and assessing the impact of possible emergencies that could affect the organization, individuals responsible for emergency management planning should consider using a variety of information sources, such as population density, seismic, and water table maps of the area. These maps can be obtained from agencies such as the National Earthquake Information Center (http://earthquake.usgs.gov/regional/neic/) and local courthouses.

Other sources of information that might be useful in the HVA process include the following:

- U.S. Department of Homeland Security: http://www.dhs.gov
- Federal Emergency Management Agency: http://fema.gov
- National Weather Service: http://www.nws.noaa.gov
- Local Emergency Planning Committee Database: http://yosemite.epa.gov/oswer/lepcdb.nsf/HomePage
- Multi-Hazard Mapping Initiative: http://gcmd.nasa.gov/records/FEMA-HazardMaps.html

References

1. Healthcare executives' role in emergency preparedness. *Healthc Exec* pp. 86–87, Mar.–Apr. 2007.
2. Lichterman J.D.: A "community as resource" strategy for disaster response. *Public Health Rep* 115:262–265, May–Jun. 2000.

Chapter 3

Developing and Maintaining an Emergency Operations Plan

Developing an emergency management plan is a lot like acquiring an insurance program for a business.[1] The hope is that plan implementation will not be needed, but if it ever is, the plan allows staff to function effectively during a disaster. A successful emergency operations plan outlines a realistic approach to ensuring that the organization's customers will experience minimal disruption in services provided. Emergency management planning should be viewed as an investment. This notion is much more common in industries beyond health care. In fact, some manufacturing firms include their disaster planning process in marketing efforts that identify competitive advantages.[1] This chapter describes how health care organizations can ensure the development of an effective "all-hazards" emergency operations plan (EOP). Sidebar 3-1 details the Joint Commission's requirements for developing and maintaining an EOP.

Developing and Maintaining an EOP

The standard requiring an EOP describes it as a document that helps guide an organization in its emergency response and recovery efforts. A successful response to an emergency relies upon planning around the management of six critical areas: communication, resources and assets, safety and security, staff responsibilities, utilities management, and patient clinical and support activities. It is important for organizations to develop a comprehensive EOP as documentation to help guide the organization in its emergency response and recovery efforts. Although the EOP can be formatted in a variety of ways, it

Sidebar 3-1.
Applicable Emergency Management Standard

The organization develops and maintains an emergency operations plan.

This standard requires the following:

- The organization develops and maintains a written emergency operations plan (EOP) that describes an "all-hazards" command structure for coordinating the six critical functions (discussed in Chapter 1) within the organization during an emergency.
- The EOP establishes an incident command structure. Hospitals and critical access hospitals must integrate this into their processes and ensure that it is consistent with the surrounding community's command structure.
- The EOP identifies to whom staff report in the organization's incident command structure.
- The EOP identifies the organization's capabilities and establishes response efforts when the organization cannot be supported by the local community for at least 96 hours in the six critical areas. Acceptable response efforts could include the following:
  - Conservation of resources (for example, alternative bathing procedures to save water)
  - Curtailment of services (for example, cancellation of elective surgeries)
  - Supplementing of resources from outside the local community
  - Total evacuation
- The EOP identifies alternative sites for care, treatment, or service that meet the needs of its patients during emergencies.

Be Prepared Tip

Structuring the Plan

Organizations should consider structuring their plans to state how the items listed in the elements of performance are met within the organization. The plan should include appropriate policies and procedures to respond to likely hazards, as defined in the hazard vulnerability analysis (HVA) described in Chapter 2.

must address these six critical areas to serve as a blueprint for managing care and safety during an emergency. The EOP replaces previous Joint Commission requirements for an emergency management plan and requires organizations to assemble the policies and procedures necessary to respond to emergencies.

Some emergencies can escalate unexpectedly and strain the organization and the entire community. An organization cannot mitigate risks, plan thoroughly, and sustain an effective response and recovery without preparing its staff and collaborating with the community, suppliers, and external response partners. Such an approach will aid the organization in developing a scalable response capability and in defining the timing and criteria for decisions that involve sheltering in place, patient transfer, facility closings, or evacuation. By describing an "all-hazards" command structure for coordinating the aforementioned six critical functions within the organization during an emergency, the plan further gives an organization the tools necessary to meet the challenges of an emergency.

The EOP itself should be a self-contained document. Some organizations might divide the document into major sections covering internal and external emergencies. These sections can begin with the all-purpose EOP, followed by subsections dealing with specific critical areas and with most-likely scenarios. In other words, how would the organization respond to specific types of events? Some organizations then further break down each subsection with entries for defined areas such as departments, formatted with a common template. This makes it easier for the average employee who is not familiar with the entire plan to figure out what he or she should do. (More about staff responsibilities can be found in Chapter 7.) Steps that could be used as a starting point to building an emergency operations plan appear in Table 3-1 and Table 3-2 (page 29).

The EOP also should be written in clear English. Staff should define all terms at the beginning and avoid using too many acronyms or abbreviations. A clearly marked glossary at the back of the document should define any acronyms or abbreviations that are used.

Incident Command Structure and Identifying Staff Reporting

The Joint Commission requires that the EOP establish an incident command system (ICS) for emergency management. For critical access hospitals and hospitals, the standard further requires that the ICS is integrated into and consistent with its community's command structure. The ICS requirement should be familiar to organizations from previous accreditation standards. A successful ICS, which should be thought of as an "all-hazards" command structure, includes the following characteristics:

- Flexibility—the structure must be adaptable to a wide variety of situations, including those that the hospital or long term care organization might not have anticipated.
- Clarity—all individuals within the organization, from clinical to clerical staff, must clearly understand their roles and responsibilities.
- Community integration—the organization's command structure must be coordinated with that of the community responders, such as emergency medical services, as well as the police and fire departments; local, state, or federal emergency management agencies; and other local health care organizations.

An ICS is a standardized incident management concept designed specifically to allow all types of emergency responders to adopt an integrated organizational structure equal to the complexity and demands of any single incident or multiple incidents without being hindered by jurisdictional boundaries.

Be Prepared Tip

Developing the Plan

Organization staff should review every issue that is addressed by the elements of performance for the Emergency Operations Plan standard because each must be covered in the plan. However, simply restating the intent in the emergency management plan is not enough. The plan should discuss the organization's method of compliance in enough detail to allow the reader to understand the process and procedures, but not so detailed as to make the plan too voluminous.

Table 3-1. Steps to Building a Customized Emergency Operations Plan

1. By conducting a hazard vulnerability analysis, as described in Chapter 2, identify the risks that can potentially affect the health care facility.
2. Add issues and assess compliance related to the Joint Commission requirements and other agencies and unlisted regulatory issues.
3. Briefly describe compliance with each requirement.
4. Cross-reference to more detailed policies and procedures.
5. Establish and document the process for information collection and evaluation.
6. Determine the content and establish the process for staff orientation and education.
7. Develop the appropriate emergency response procedures.
8. Identify appropriate performance monitors based on actual or potential risk.
9. Establish the process for annual evaluation of the plan.

Source: Joint Commission Resources: *Guide to Emergency Management Planning in Health Care.* Oakbrook Terrace, IL: Joint Commission on Accreditation of Healthcare Organizations, 2002.

Table 3-2. Developing a Disaster Plan

The Agency for Healthcare Research and Quality (AHRQ) recommends the following steps for developing a disaster plan:

1. Assemble an interdisciplinary team of key stakeholders for disaster planning.
2. Review current resources, strengths, and weaknesses.
3. Develop a detailed written disaster response plan.
4. Disseminate and practice the plan through education and drills.
5. Evaluate the adequacy of knowledge, skills, and resources.
6. Revise the plan based on objective data and lessons learned.
7. Modify education and training as needed to target areas of weakness.
8. Continuously repeat these steps.

Key components of the plan, the AHRQ says, should include an incident command system, system integration, logistics, security, clinical care, human resources, and public relations.

Source: Agency for Healthcare Research and Quality (AHRQ): *Bioterrorism and Health System Preparedness: Disaster Planning Drills and Readiness Assessment.* Rockville, MD: AHRQ, Jan. 2004.

Emergency Operations Plan Checklist

- Surveillance and epidemiological process
- Identification of command structure and authorized personnel
- Notification process
- Activation in stages (alert, standby, callout, stand-down)
- Response plan by department
- Command center location, equipment, staffing, and alternative locations
- Communications systems if all usual lines and methods fail (radios, runners, and so forth)
- Local/regional coordination plan
- Security plan to control access and egress
- Internal traffic flow and control
- Media management and response
- Reception of casualties and victims (identification, triage, stabilization, admission or transfer, transport)
- Meeting care/communication needs of specific populations (non-English-speaking, elderly, pediatric)
- Volunteer plan
- Information sharing plans
- Facility evacuation
- Relocation of care recipients and staff
- Decontamination, isolation, or quarantine
- Assessment of equipment, facility, and laboratory supplies
- Availability of pharmaceuticals

Be Prepared Tip

Incident Command System Structure

The incident command system (ICS) typically puts one individual (the incident commander) in charge of the emergency and decision-making process. Other positions or roles in an ICS, depending on the size and complexity of the organization, include public information officer, safety and security officer, liaison officer, liaison chief, planning chief, finance chief, and operations chief. Which of these positions is activated depends on the extent and type of the emergency encountered.

An "All-Hazards" Command Structure

An effective command system takes an "all-hazards" approach, with the following characteristics:

- A flexible structure for response to a variety of emergencies
- Clear delineation of staff roles and responsibilities
- A predictable chain of command
- Accountability for staff involved
- Prioritized response checklists
- The use of common terminology to reduce miscommunication
- The ability to be integrated into a communitywide plan

Source: Joint Commission Resources: *Are You Prepared? Hospital Emergency Management Guidebook.* Oakbrook Terrace, IL: Joint Commission on Accreditation of Healthcare Organizations, 2006.

In the early 1970s ICS was developed to manage rapidly moving wildfires and to address the following problems[2]:

- Too many people reporting to one supervisor
- Different emergency response organization structures
- Lack of reliable incident information
- Inadequate and incompatible communications
- Lack of structure for coordinated planning among agencies
- Unclear lines of authority
- Terminology differences among agencies
- Unclear or unspecified incident objectives

Although the EOP standard does not require a specific system, community integration itself is considered critical. Several models exist, including the National Incident Management System (NIMS), the Hospital Incident Command System (HICS), and the Fire Service Incident Command System. (*See* Figure 3-1 (pages 31–35) and Sidebar 3-2 (pages 36–38) and the scenario presented within it for more information on HICS and NIMS.) The HICS is probably the most well-known command structure model used in health care organizations throughout the country, defining staff responsibilities and reporting channels and using common terminology.

One of the reasons for the popularity of the HICS is its flexibility. This system provides a temporary organizational structure that enables individuals to be rotated into various roles as time and circumstances dictate. The command staff includes the incident commander, liaison officer, public information officer, safety officer, and medical technical specialist. The medical technical specialist is a role that can be filled depending on the type of event, such as a specialist in pediatric or biological or infectious disease. Beyond the command staff, the HICS further defines roles related to operations, planning, logistics, and finance/operations.

The HICS's use of an organizational chart is useful in clearly delineating the roles and responsibilities of staff members and leaders during an emergency. In addition, the HICS can be easily integrated into an organization's EOP and fits well with communitywide emergency efforts because of its standardization of roles and use of common terminology.

It is worth noting that no fixed model, whether it is the HICS, the NIMS, or another model, should be adopted in totality without intensive consultation with the involved community agencies. Modifications will undoubtedly be required to adapt to the given health care organization.

For any ICS to be successfully implemented, staff must understand to whom they report. This is important because emergency situations are likely to result in a reporting structure different than what staff are accustomed to, and staff must be not only ready to work, but cooperative in working toward a common goal.

Figure 3-1. Hospital Incident Command System Examples

This Hospital Incident Command System (HICS) incident management team chart depicts the hospital command functions that have been identified and represents how authority and responsibility are distributed within the incident management team.

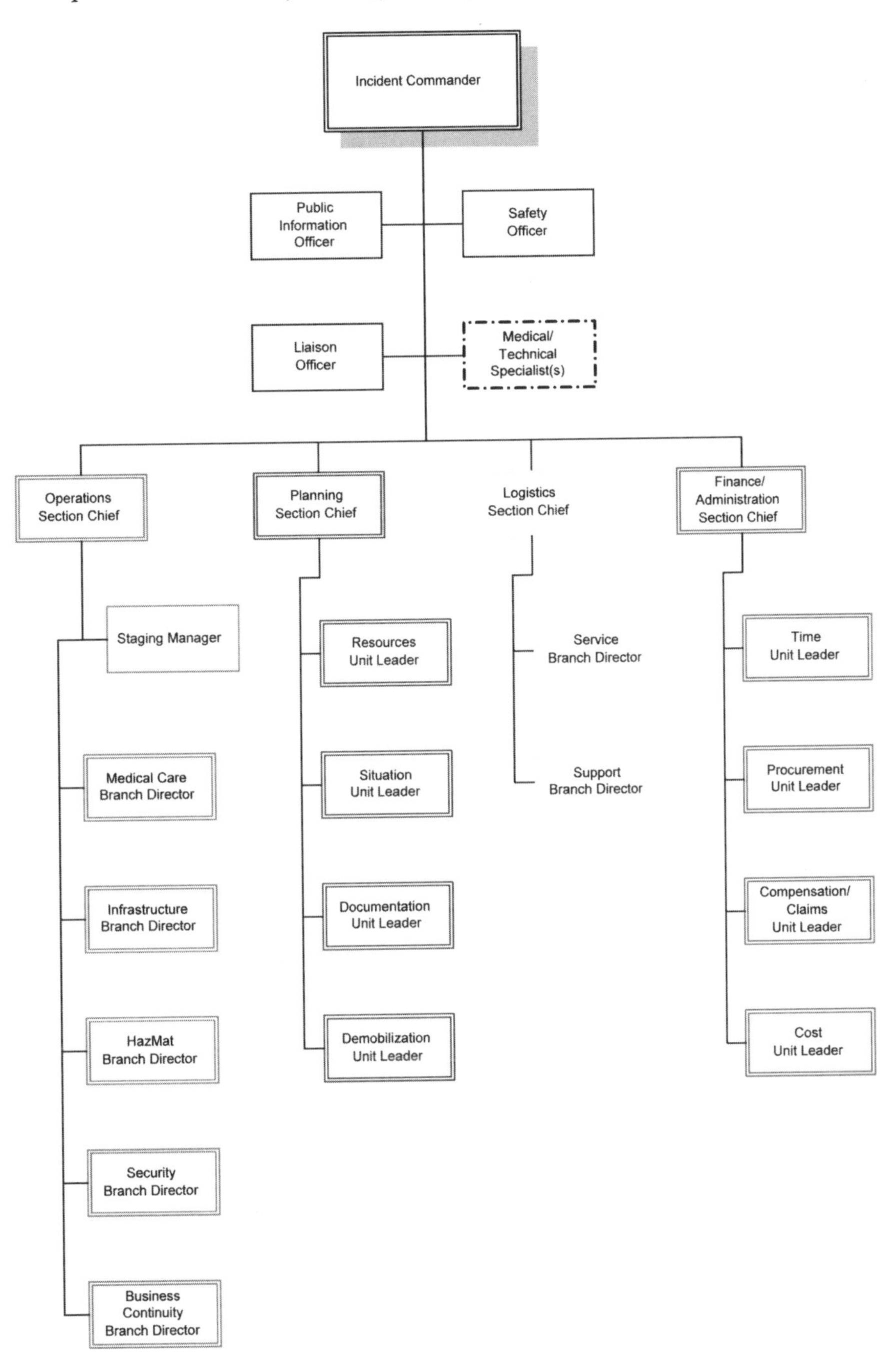

Source: Reprinted from HICS IV "Hospital Incident Command Guidebook," Aug. 2006. California Emergency Medical Services Authority. Available online at http://www.emsa.ca.gov/Dms2/download.htm.

(continued)

Figure 3-1. Hospital Incident Command System Examples, *continued*

This Job Action Sheet (JAS) is an incident management tool designed to familiarize the user with critical aspects of the Incident Commander position. There are many JASs listed within the HICS guidebook, distributed among the categories of "Command," "Medical/Technical Specialists," "Operations," Planning," "Logistics," and "Finance/Administration."

Job Action Sheet　　COMMAND

INCIDENT COMMANDER

Mission: Organize and direct the Hospital Command Center (HCC). Give overall strategic direction for hospital incident management and support activities, including emergency response and recovery. Authorize total facility evacuation if warranted.

Date: ________ Start: _______ End: _______ Position Assigned to: ____________________

Signature: ______________________________________ Initial: __________

Hospital Command Center (HCC) Location: ________________ Telephone: ____________

Fax: ________________ Other Contact Info: ____________ Radio Title: ____________

Immediate (Operational Period 0-2 Hours)	Time	Initial
Assume role of Incident Commander and activate the Hospital Incident Command System (HICS).		
Read this entire Job Action Sheet and put on position identification.		
Notify your usual supervisor and the hospital CEO, or designee, of the incident, activation of HICS and your HICS assignment.		
Initiate the Incident Briefing Form (HICS Form 201) and include the following information: • Nature of the problem (incident type, victim count, injury/illness type, etc.) • Safety of staff, patients and visitors • Risks to personnel and need for protective equipment • Risks to the facility • Need for decontamination • Estimated duration of incident • Need for modifying daily operations • HICS team required to manage the incident • Need to open up the HCC • Overall community response actions being taken • Status of local, county, and state Emergency Operations Centers (EOC)		
Contact hospital operator and initiate hospital's emergency operations plan.		
Determine need for and appropriately appoint Command Staff and Section Chiefs, or Branch/Unit/Team leaders and Medical/Technical Specialists as needed; distribute corresponding Job Action Sheets and position identification. Assign or complete the Branch Assignment List (HICS Form 204), as appropriate.		
Brief all appointed staff of the nature of the problem, immediate critical issues and initial plan of action. Designate time for next briefing.		
Assign one of more clerical personnel from current staffing or make a request for staff to the Labor Pool and Credentialing Unit Leader, if activated, to function as the HCC recorder(s).		
Distribute the Section Personnel Time Sheet (HICS Form 252) to Command Staff and Medical/Technical Specialist assigned to Command, and ensure time is recorded appropriately. Submit the Section Personnel Time Sheet to the Finance/Administration Section's Time Unit Leader at the completion of a shift or at the end of each operational period.		
Initiate the Incident Action Plan Safety Analysis (HICS Form 261) to document hazards and define mitigation.		

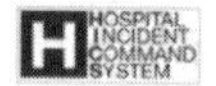

August 2006

(continued)

Figure 3-1. Hospital Incident Command System Examples, *continued*

Job Action Sheet

Command
INCIDENT COMMANDER
Page 2

Immediate (Operational Period 0-2 Hours)	**Time**	**Initial**
Receive status reports from and develop an Incident Action Plan with Section Chiefs and Command Staff to determine appropriate response and recovery levels. During initial briefing/status reports, discover the following: • If applicable, receive initial facility damage survey report from Logistics Section Chief and evaluate the need for evacuation. • If applicable, obtain patient census and status from Planning Section Chief, and request a hospital-wide projection report for 4, 8, 12, 24 & 48 hours from time of incident onset. Adjust projections as necessary. • Identify the operational period and HCC shift change. • If additional beds are needed, authorize a patient prioritization assessment for the purposes of designating appropriate early discharge. • Ensure that appropriate contact with outside agencies has been established and facility status and resource information provided through the Liaison Officer. • Seek information from Section Chiefs regarding current "on-hand" resources of medical equipment, supplies, medications, food, and water as indicated by the incident. • Review security and facility surge capacity and capability plans as appropriate.		
Document all key activities, actions, and decisions in an Operational Log (HICS Form 214) on a continual basis.		
Document all communications (internal and external) on an Incident Message Form (HICS Form 213). Provide a copy of the Incident Message Form to the Documentation Unit.		

Intermediate (Operational Period 2-12 Hours)	**Time**	**Initial**
Authorize resources as needed or requested by Command Staff.		
Designate regular briefings with Command Staff/Section Chiefs to identify and plan for: • Update of current situation/response and status of other area hospitals, emergency management/local emergency operation centers, and public health officials and other community response agencies • Deploying a Liaison Officer to local EOC • Deploying a PIO to the local Joint Information Center • Critical facility and patient care issues • Hospital operational support issues • Risk communication and situation updates to staff • Implementation of hospital surge capacity and capability plans • Ensure patient tracking system established and linked with appropriate outside agencies and/or local EOC • Family Support Center operations • Public information, risk communication and education needs • Appropriate use and activation of safety practices and procedures • Enhanced staff protection measures as appropriate • Public information and education needs • Media relations and briefings • Staff and family support • Development, review, and/or revision of the Incident Action Plan, or elements of the Incident Action Plan		
Oversee and approve revision of the Incident Action Plan developed by the Planning Section Chief. Ensure that the approved plan is communicated to all Command Staff and Section Chiefs.		
Communicate facility and incident status and the Incident Action Plan to CEO or designee, or to other executives and/or Board of Directors members on a need-to-know basis.		

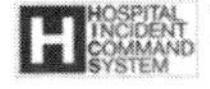

August 2006

(continued)

Figure 3-1. Hospital Incident Command System Examples, *continued*

Job Action Sheet

Command
INCIDENT COMMANDER
Page 3

Extended (Operational Period Beyond 12 Hours)	**Time**	**Initial**
Ensure staff, patient, and media briefings are being conducted regularly.		
Review and revise the Incident Action Plan Safety Analysis (HICS Form 261) and implement correction or mitigation strategies.		
Evaluate/re-evaluate need for deploying a Liaison Officer to the local EOC.		
Evaluate/re-evaluate need for deploying a PIO to the local Joint Information Center.		
Ensure incident action planning for each operational period and a reporting of the Incident Action Plan at each shift change and briefing.		
Evaluate overall hospital operational status, and ensure critical issues are addressed.		
Review /revise the Incident Action Plan with the Planning Section Chief for each operational period.		
Ensure continued communications with local, regional, and state response coordination centers and other HCCs through the Liaison Officer and others.		
Ensure your physical readiness, and that of the Command Staff and Section Chiefs, through proper nutrition, water intake, rest periods and relief, and stress management techniques.		
Observe all staff and volunteers for signs of stress and inappropriate behavior. Report concerns to the Employee Health & Well-Being Unit Leader.		
Upon shift change, brief your replacement on the status of all ongoing operations, critical issues, relevant incident information and Incident Action Plan for the next operational period.		

Demobilization/System Recovery	**Time**	**Initial**
Assess the plan developed by the Demobilization Unit Leader and approved by the Planning Section Chief for the gradual demobilization of the HCC and emergency operations according to the progression of the incident and facility/hospital status. Demobilize positions in the HCC and return personnel to their normal jobs as appropriate until the incident is resolved and there is a return to normal operations. • Briefing staff, administration, and Board of Directors • Approve announcement of "ALL CLEAR" when incident is no longer a critical safety threat or can be managed using normal hospital operations • Ensure outside agencies are aware of status change • Declare hospital/facility safety		
Ensure demobilization of the HCC and restocking of supplies, as appropriate including: • Return of borrowed equipment to appropriate location • Replacement of broken or lost items • Cleaning of HCC and facility • Restock of HCC supplies and equipment; • Environmental clean-up as warranted		
Ensure that after-action activities are coordinated and completed including: • Collection of all HCC documentation by the Planning Section Chief • Coordination and submission of response and recovery costs, and reimbursement documentation by the Finance/Administration and Planning Section Chiefs • Conduct of staff debriefings to identify accomplishments, response and improvement issues • Identify needed revisions to the Emergency Management Plan, Emergency		

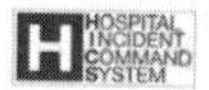

August 2006

(continued)

Figure 3-1. Hospital Incident Command System Examples, *continued*

Job Action Sheet

Command
INCIDENT COMMANDER
Page 4

Demobilization/System Recovery	Time	Initial
Operations Plan, Job Action Sheets, operational procedures, records, and/or other related items • Writing the facility/hospital After Action Report and Improvement Plan • Participation in external (community and governmental) meetings and other post-incident discussion and after-action activities • Post-incident media briefings and facility/hospital status updates • Post-incident public education and information • Stress management activities and services for staff		

Documents/Tools

- Incident Action Plan
- HICS Form 201 – Incident Briefing Form
- HICS Form 204 – Branch Assignment List
- HICS Form 207 – Incident Management Team Chart
- HICS Form 213 – Incident Message Form
- HICS Form 214 – Operational Log
- HICS Form 252 – Section Personnel Time Sheet
- HICS Form 261 – Incident Action Plan Safety Analysis
- Hospital emergency operations plan and other plans as cited in the JAS
- Hospital organization chart
- Hospital telephone directory
- Radio/satellite phone

Source: Reprinted from HICS IV "Hospital Incident Command Guidebook" ("Appendix C Materials—Job Action Sheets"), Aug. 2006. California Emergency Medical Services Authority. Available online at http://www.emsa.cahwnet.gov./hics/job_action_sheets.asp.

Be Prepared Tip

Making the Hospital Incident Command System Work

Implementing the Hospital Incident Command System does not necessarily ensure that a hospital will be able to effectively respond to a mass-casualty incident; that requires collaboration between hospital teams, leadership, and external agencies locally and nationally. Teams require flawless communication and coordination to maintain the awareness required to manage these complex events.

Sidebar 3-2.

Using the National Incident Management System and the Hospital Incident Command System to Navigate the Emergency Management Process

Emergency management is not something that can be done "on the fly." To be effective at emergency response, organizations must use an approach that is planned and structured, yet flexible and scalable. Not only does this make common business sense, but federal, state, and local governments, as well as accrediting agencies, such as The Joint Commission, require it. Creating an emergency management program that encompasses an "all-hazards" approach can be daunting for some organizations. To help with this process, organizations might wish to seek compliance with an existing emergency management system. Two of the most common systems are the National Incident Management System (NIMS) and the Hospital Incident Command System (HICS).

What Is the NIMS?

In 2004, through a presidential declaration, the NIMS was created. The NIMS is intended to be an umbrella approach for unifying local, state, and federal responses to emergencies. The system is designed to promote collaboration, integration, and interoperability and ultimately lead to better responses to emergencies by communities throughout the United States.

The NIMS was not specifically designed for hospitals and health care systems; however, several such organizations have pursued NIMS implementation since 2004. In 2006 the NIMS Integration Center (NIC), in collaboration with the Department of Health and Human Services (HHS), released a document targeted to hospitals and health care systems, *NIMS Implementation Activities for Hospitals and Healthcare Systems.*[1]

"Hospitals and health care systems are not required by the government to comply with NIMS. However, health care organizations seeking federal funding from the Health Resources and Services Administration (HRSA) must comply with NIMS," says Jerry Gervais, C.H.S.P., C.H.F.M., associate director, Standards Interpretation Group, The Joint Commission. The HRSA required hospitals and other health care organizations seeking funding to complete NIMS implementation before August 31, 2007.

Organizations must implement 17 elements to be compliant with the NIMS. These elements address the following seven principal topic areas:

1. Organizational adoption
2. Command and management
3. Preparedness planning
4. Preparedness training
5. Preparedness exercises
6. Resource management
7. Communication and information management

The previously mentioned HHS implementation document gives background, implementation guidance, implementation examples, and references for each of these health care–focused elements.

Ultimately, the implementation of the 17 activities is designed to enhance the relationship between hospitals and their respective local government, public health, and other emergency response agencies. According to the NIC, "Hospitals and health care systems are strongly encouraged to coordinate with local public health agencies to work through these implementation activities."[1] For more information on the NIMS, organizations can go to http://www.fema.gov/emergency/nims/nims_compliance.shtm.

What Is the HICS?

The HICS, revised in August 2006, is an incident management system that assists hospitals in improving their emergency management planning, response, and recovery capabilities for both unplanned and planned events. The principles embodied in the HICS are applicable to both emergent and nonemergent incidents. (The HICS was formerly called the Hospital Emergency Incident Command System [HEICS]; however, due to its applicability to both emergency and nonemergency events, the word *emergency* was dropped from the original name.)

The HICS is a methodology for using an incident command system (ICS) in a hospital/health care environment. It was redesigned in 2006 to parallel the NIMS program.

(continued)

Sidebar 3-2, *continued*

Using the National Incident Management System and the Hospital Incident Command System to Navigate the Emergency Management Process

HICS materials include a variety of useful emergency management tools, including the following:

- A guidebook to the HICS
- Incident command practices
- HICS implementation and utilization considerations
- Incident planning guides
- Job action sheets (JAS) for each incident management team position
- Documentation forms
- Electronic slideshow education modules

"There are also incident response guides (IRGs) that serve as emergency management brain teasers for incident commanders and staff," says Craig DeAtley, director of the Institute for Public Health Emergency Readiness at the Washington Hospital Center in Washington, D.C., and co-project manager for the HICS IV project, sponsored by the California Emergency Management Services Authority (EMSA). "The IRGs are based on 14 external and 13 internal emergency scenarios and can be used to help organizations train and drill for emergencies." External drills focus on topics such as plague and anthrax, and internal drills include such topics as child abduction, fire, and utility loss. (*See* the box at right for an example of an external scenario.)

It is important to note that the HICS is not a template for a hospital emergency management plan, nor is it a hospital emergency operations plan. It is an emergency management system that focuses on the ICS. All HICS materials are posted on the California EMSA Web site (http://www.emsa.ca.gov) and are available for download at no cost. The national work group that created HICS Education and Training recently launched a Web site (http://www.hicscenter.org) as a repository for all HICS materials. "This Web site helps us share lessons learned from organizations using HICS and also provides access to the people who designed the HICS for individuals with questions," says DeAtley. "We have also created an 8-hour introductory training to HICS and a 16-hour train-the-trainer course."

External Drill Scenario: Anthrax Exposure

The following is an example of an external scenario provided by the HICS.

Urban City is a metropolis with a large commuter workforce with major hubs where large numbers of commuters congregate while waiting for connections. Recently, Urban City has been experiencing an early influenza season, with more than usual numbers of people becoming ill with colds and flu.

One weekday, the Universal Adversary terrorist group disburses aerosol anthrax among the commuters using a concealed improvising spray device. The commuters do not notice the fine aerosol hanging in the air around them.

Twelve hours post-release, patients within and outside of Urban City present to emergency departments with influenza-illness-like complaints and symptoms. Many are seen and discharged, whereas a few are serious enough to require admission. Eighteen hours post-release, with large numbers of patients overwhelming emergency departments and clinics, and with multiple fatalities, a diagnosis of respiratory anthrax is made in several hospitals in the area. Local public health departments determine that the cases shared common commute locations and issue a case definition and alert to health care providers. Law enforcement and the Centers for Disease Control and Prevention are notified.

Source: California Emergency Medical Services Authority: *Hospital Incident Command System—External Scenarios.* http://www.emsa.ca.gov/hics/external_scenarios.asp (accessed Feb. 10, 2008).

How Are the HICS and the NIMS Related?

"Although HICS is not required for federal funding, it is a helpful tool for organizations seeking NIMS compliance or compliance with Joint Commission standards," says DeAtley. Although HICS is consistent and compatible with NIMS

(continued)

Sidebar 3-2, *continued*

Using the National Incident Management System and the Hospital Incident Command System to Navigate the Emergency Management Process

principles, by itself it will not result in a hospital being totally compliant with all NIMS activities. For example, the NIMS has specific training requirements for individuals assuming an incident command management position and for other individuals involved in incident command. "While HICS does not require specific education, the program does provide education modules that explain all the information found in the HICS package," says DeAtley. In addition, the previously mentioned HICS introductory training and train-the-trainer courses are designed to cover most of the specific course listings found in the NIMS guidance document. "HICS is not intended to address all 17 NIMS activity areas," says DeAtley. "But it does support NIMS practices and is a designed program that provides health care organizations with a comprehensive, adaptable, scalable, and flexible approach to incident command. Plus, many organizations are already using the HEICS system and have a head start on complying with HICS." Key difference from the HEICS include the incident management team chart with updated and expanded JAS, NIMS/HICS–compliant forms for documentation, hazard-specific planning and operational guidance, and information for addressing the NIMS.[2]

The HICS, The NIMS, and Joint Commission Standards

Both the HICS and the NIMS can help organizations comply with the Joint Commission's emergency management standards. "The Joint Commission standards relating to emergency management require organizations to take an 'all-hazards' approach to managing emergencies, including establishing an 'all-hazards' command structure. Both the HICS and NIMS help organizations establish such a structure," says Gervais. Although the HICS and the NIMS can be used to comply with many of the Joint Commission requirements, compliance with the HICS or the NIMS does not automatically mean compliance with Joint Commission requirements found in the Emergency Operations Plan standard. The Joint Commission standards offer a framework for effective emergency management, and each organization must tailor an effective program for emergency management within that framework.

References

1. Federal Emergency Management Agency: NIMS implementation activities for hospitals and healthcare systems. *NIMS Alert,* Sep. 12, 2006.
2. California Emergency Management Services Authority: *California EMSA Releases HICS Guide.* Oct. 19, 2006.

Source: Reprinted from Joint Commission Resources: Managing an emergency. *Environment of Care News* 10:5, May 2007.

Be Prepared Tip

Readying the Command Post

At a minimum, the command post should have emergency power and be stocked with cellular phones, flashlights, battery-powered lamps, portable radios, telephones, computer network hookups, and detailed building plans. It is not necessary for all this equipment to be physically located in the command post, but it should be easy to find and transport there when needed. There should also be a list in the command post of critical telephone, pager, and fax numbers.

The EOP should state that the organization operates under an ICS that is coordinated with the community, along with a few details about the process and a cross-reference to the policy and/or procedure for doing so. The EOP also should identify to whom staff report in the organization's incident command structure. Early steps in coping with most emergencies and putting an EOP into place are notifying key staff and setting up the command post. The plan must clearly spell out the following:

- Who is the responsible individual to be contacted
- All areas of responsibility
- The circumstances under which the plan is to be activated and by whom
- Who is initially in charge

During business hours, for example, the administrative offices of Medicare-/Medicaid-based long term care organizations or the emergency departments of hospitals most often get calls. At other times, in a rapidly developing incident, the first person notified is the in-house nursing supervisor, the emergency department supervisor, or the administrator on call. In more slowly evolving incidents, the CEO or his or her designee is the first to be contacted by the administrative offices. If the CEO is not the initial activator of the plan, then the plan should describe what actions the activator should take and how to ultimately transfer to the CEO or designee at the command post. It is important to specify the chain of notification in the plan, including what key staff must be notified at the onset of an emergency, and to review the contact numbers periodically. Because outgoing communications might become jammed by a flood of incoming phone calls, even when the phone system is not directly affected by the emergency, there should be a contingency plan for other ways to reach people. (Establishing emergency communications strategies is discussed in detail in Chapter 4.)

The individual in charge of the organization's central command site must be in regular communication with first response teams at the site of the emergency. This gives the organization a greater understanding of the magnitude of the emergency and helps the command site know if, when, and how many patients are leaving the emergency site for treatment at the facility, as well as the severity of any injuries.

The command post needs to be in a predesignated area of the health care organization, and it is also a good idea to identify an alternative site in case the emergency affects the command post itself or prevents access to it. The plan should state who is responsible for delivering equipment to the command post and setting it up. Some suggested numbers to have on hand are listed in Table 3-3 (page 40).

Staff essential to the health care organization's operation should be assigned to the command post. Together, members of this group will oversee carrying out the EOP. Depending on the size of the organization and the number of available resources, this group usually includes the CEO or director, chief operating officer, chief financial officers, chief of the medical staff, chief nursing officer, director of nursing, director of plant operations, media/marketing director, and security chief. Secretarial assistance also might be useful in the command post. Sidebar 3-3 (page 40) provides information about how to develop and maintain an EOP and an ICS.

Initiating and Terminating Response and Recovery Phases

The EOP should be specific in describing the processes for initiating and terminating the response and recovery phases of emergency management, including who has the authority to activate the phases and how the phases are to be activated. The Joint Commission emphasizes these two aspects of emergency management in the EOP standard. Being specific in how the response phase begins and ends is critical because the *response* refers to the actual emergency management of treating victims, reducing impact to the organization, and controlling the negative effects of the emergency situation(s). The *recovery* phase is likewise important because it means that the organization is moving back to normal operations. Again, in detailing initiation and termination of response and recovery phases, the EOP should address the six critical areas of emergency management (communication, resources and assets, safety and security, staff responsibilities, utilities management, and patient clinical and support activities).

Going It Alone for 96 Hours

One of the new emergency management requirements relates to the need to plan for what an organization will do when the community cannot assist or support it. Large-scale disasters such as the terrorist attacks of 2001 and Hurricane Katrina on the Gulf Coast demonstrated how an event can cripple a region and leave health care organizations on their own. Creating a detailed EOP in the face of uncertain resource support is a daunting challenge.

The EOP standard requires that the EOP identify the organization's capabilities and establish response efforts when the organization cannot be supported by the local community for at least

Table 3-3. Telephone Numbers to Have in the Command Post

- Contact numbers for all departments
  - Telephone
  - Fax
- Contact numbers for key staff
  - Home phone
  - Pager
  - Fax
  - Next-of-kin notification
- Pay phones in the facility and their locations
- Elevator telephones
- Neighboring health care organizations
- Regional contacts
  - Police
  - Fire department
  - Public/state health department
  - National Guard
  - Civil defense
  - Red Cross
  - Television stations, radio stations, and print media
  - State and county emergency operations centers
  - Essential vendors (linen, food, fuel, etc.)
  - Utility companies
  - Blood banks
  - Ambulance services
  - Coroner's office
  - Nursing registry
  - County medical society
  - Funeral homes
  - Pharmacies

Source: Joint Commission Resources: *Guide to Emergency Management Planning in Health Care.* Oakbrook Terrace, IL: Joint Commission on Accreditation of Healthcare Organizations, 2002.

Sidebar 3-3.

Developing and Maintaining an Emergency Operations Plan and an Incident Command System

Whereas the standard requiring the management of the consequences of emergencies discusses the planning aspect of emergency management, the EOP standard addresses an organization's response. The standard requires organizations to develop and maintain an Emergency Operations Plan (EOP). This is a document to help guide an organization in its emergency response and recovery efforts and should include a description of the organization's incident command system (ICS).

"An ICS at a fundamental level helps organizations identify who is in charge during an emergency and which individuals will carry out the decisions of the individual in charge," says James Augustine, M.D., an emergency medicine physician at Emory University in Atlanta. Augustine serves as the American College of Emergency Physicians liaison to the Joint Commission's Hospital Professional and Technical Advisory Committee and thus had input into the development of the revised emergency management standards. "An ICS does not need to be rigid, but everyone in an organization should understand the basic principles of the ICS and how it applies on a day-to-day basis. If this basic understanding exists, then staff can scale up response efforts when necessary."

Peter Brewster, director of education and training for the Emergency Management Strategic Healthcare Group, a part of the U.S. Department of Veterans Affairs, points out that one important aspect of emergency response addressed in the new standards is the focus on health care organization sustainability. "Organizations must understand how they will continue operations even when the community cannot support them," he says. Specifically, within the EOP, an organization must understand how it would respond to an emergency in which community support is unavailable for 96 hours.

"It is important to realize that an appropriate response may involve closing or evacuating the health care organization after a certain period," explains John Fishbeck, R.A., associate director, Division of Standards and Survey Methods, The Joint Commission. "For example, if an organization determines it has enough fuel and supplies to last for 48 hours, then it knows it can effectively continue operations for that time period. However, the organization also must realize that after 48 hours without community support, it must either evacuate or discharge patients. This is something that should be considered and planned for."

Source: Reprinted from Joint Commission Resources: Revised emergency management standards for 2008. *Environment of Care News* 10:8, Aug. 2007.

Ten Weaknesses in Emergency Operations Plans

1. Lack of critical information
2. Not flexible enough
3. Do not address communication issues broadly or in enough detail
4. Do not contain enough multidisciplinary input
5. Do not contain adaptable forms for managing information
6. Do not consider enough scenarios (or enough hazard vulnerabilities)
7. Poorly document incidents
8. Do not include troubleshooting tools
9. Lack alarm points signaling that critical supplies are running low
10. Have not undergone a detailed review with local agencies and do not consider community linkages or processes

Source: Bruce C.: Troubleshooting your top ten weaknesses in emergency preparedness plans. *Environment of Care News* 3(2):11, 2000.

96 hours. Acceptable response efforts include conserving resources or supplementing them from beyond the affected area, curtailing some services, or evacuating the facility. In other words, hospitals and long term care organizations must consider how they will address communication, resources and assets, safety and security, staff responsibilities, utilities management, and patient clinical and support activities (see the standards discussion in Chapters 4 through 9) over a four-day period if an emergency leaves them without any outside assistance.

If an organization chooses to stay, it must have plans to be self-sufficient for 96 hours. If this is not possible, then the organization should have plans in place to evacuate after a predetermined period. For example, an organization might determine that it can be self-sufficient during an emergency for 48 hours, after which point it will initiate evacuation procedures. However, the organization should also make plans so that its evacuation can be supported 48 hours after the start of an emergency. If the organization begins evacuating at 48 hours and the rest of the community has evacuated after 12 hours, the health care organization might run into significant problems.[3]

Identifying Alternative Care Sites

The last requirement for the standard under discussion in this chapter is one that has long existed in emergency standards: identifying alternative sites for care that meet the needs of patients during emergencies. When a health care organization's facility cannot support adequate patient care, or if it becomes unusable, then the organization must initiate processes for establishing an alternative care site(s) that has the capabilities to meet patient needs.

Some issues to consider when choosing an alternative care site include the following:

- How patients, staff, and equipment will be moved
- How medical records and medications will be moved
- How patients will be tracked to, within, and from the site
- How interfacility communication will occur

It might be useful to maintain a list of neighboring health care organizations that includes their staffing and equipment capabilities. The list should start with the closest facility and end with the one that is farthest away. These relationships should be defined and spelled out, in detail, in the EOP prior to a disaster.

Hospitals and long term care organizations should consider establishing prearranged mutual aid agreements with other local or area institutes to serve as alternative care sites. State hospital or nursing home associations, local emergency planning committees, or other similar groups might be able to assist in coordinating such agreements. The memorandum of understanding, though, is only a starting point, as it requires additional planning and practice to be functional during an emergency.

Cooperative planning among health care organizations also should include the following:

- Essential elements of the command structures and control centers for emergency response
- Names, roles, and telephone numbers of individuals in the command structures
- Resources and assets that could potentially be shared or pooled in an emergency response (*see* the discussion in Chapter 5)

CASE EXAMPLE:
LOUISIANA HOSPITAL FACES A WEEK ALONE AFTER HURRICANE KATRINA

East Jefferson General Hospital (EJGH) in Metairie, Louisiana, had a solid disaster plan in place. However, it was not sufficient for a disaster on the scale of Hurricane Katrina. The plan, which was designed for a disaster lasting two to three days, became irrelevant just as the crisis was getting started. However, this is not to say that the plan was not valuable.

"Some might say that our disaster plan didn't work," says Donald Chenoweth, EJGH's chief information officer. "But in a lot of ways, it still did. Because we had put a lot of work into developing the plan, there was a level of discipline that the emergency team had. Even though we weren't able to use some of the specific details of the plan, we knew what to bring in, we knew what to worry about, we knew what we had to get fixed first. That adaptability and the ability to work well under significant pressure came from our plan."

With water lapping at the back door, the generator that powered the air-conditioning having gone out, and no phone or Internet access, EJGH was effectively isolated from the rest of the city for about a week. "The biggest concern was that we didn't know how long it was going to be like that," Chenoweth says. "Fortunately, we have a very smart and flexible staff."

To regain Internet access, EJGH staff located a single dial-up line that was still working because it went through Baton Rouge instead of New Orleans. They connected PCs to it and set up some free, Web-based e-mail accounts. They also realized that although local cell phone service was down, a few phones that had exchanges outside the local area codes were occasionally working—and although voice service was sporadic, text messaging was usually operating normally.

With these simple communication methods, staff were able to communicate with friends, family, and coworkers; make contact with federal, state, and local disaster efforts; and order food, water, and medical supplies for the more than 3,000 patients, staff, and evacuees in the facility.

Through a great deal of effort and ingenuity (and some good fortune, Chenoweth says), EJGH was able to receive patients again just one week after the storm began. Many of these new patients included Hurricane Katrina survivors and emergency workers.

Since then, EJGH has revised its disaster plan significantly. "Our old disaster plan was built around being able to recover equipment and get systems back up and running so that we can continue to treat patients, but our equipment was fine," Chenoweth says. "What happened was that we became isolated and didn't have power, and nobody thought that would take place."

Because the biggest problem EJGH saw during the hurricane was the failure of its communication methods, that was the focus of revisions to the plan, Chenoweth says. "We had a lot of lines, but they all went down. We had backup cell phones, but the only ones that were working were the ones with phone numbers from out-of-state locations, and we found that out by accident.

"The new plan calls for high-speed Internet access and phones to be connected through a satellite. If we'd had that during Katrina, we would have had plenty of ability to communicate," says Chenoweth. "Not being able to contact anyone outside the hospital was nerve-wracking, but now we're modifying our plan to take care of that."

Source: Joint Commission Resources: *Safer Emergency Care: Strategies and Solutions.* Oakbrook Terrace, IL: Joint Commission on Accreditation of Healthcare Organizations, 2007, p. 87.

Be Prepared Tip

Agency for Healthcare Research and Quality Tool for Alternative Care Sites

The Agency for Healthcare Research and Quality (AHRQ) has released a tool to quickly locate alternative care sites in the event that hospitals are overwhelmed by patients due to a bioterrorist attack or other public health emergency. The tool, produced by AHRQ partner Denver Health Medical Center, allows regional emergency planners to locate and rank potential alternative sites, such as stadiums, schools, recreation centers, motels, and other venues, based on whether they have such resources as adequate ventilation, plumbing, toilet facilities, communication lines, and food service areas. The tool lists about 30 attributes in all. The spreadsheet, which also addresses necessary equipment, supplies, staffing considerations, and coordination with local agencies to ensure that potential sites have not been designated for another use, is available at AHRQ's Web site at http://www.ahrq.gov.

Non–health care organization sites also should be considered as potential alternative care sites. These could include schools, college dormitories, libraries, recreation centers, sports stadiums, military armories, closed hospitals, places of worship, and hotels. Even large corporate buildings might have spaces that could serve as areas to deliver care or as discharge centers. Health care orga-nizations should coordinate with other local agencies, however, to ensure that potential sites have not been designated for another use.

There are many factors to consider when selecting an alternative care site. Some might be less or more important, depending on the type of emergency at hand and the time of year that the emergency occurs. For example, ventilation might be less of an issue if victims do not have to be isolated or decontaminated. Heating is not as important if the event occurs in the summer or in a warm part of the country. Table 3-4 (page 44) provides a list of possible alternative care sites that organizations might wish to consider. Among the factors to consider when selecting an alternative care site are the following[4]:

- Ability to lock down the facility
- Adequate building security personnel
- Adequate lighting
- Air-conditioning/ventilation
- Area for equipment storage
- Biohazard and other waste disposal
- Communications capability
- Door size adequate for gurneys
- Electrical power with backup
- Family areas
- Flood supply/preparation area
- Floor and walls adequate
- Heating
- Laboratory/specimen handling areas
- Laundry area
- Loading dock
- Oxygen delivery ability, compressed medical air, and suction availability
- Parking for staff/visitors
- Patient decontamination areas
- Pharmacy areas
- Proximity to hospital/long term care facility
- Toilet facilities/showers/waste
- Two-way radio capability
- Water supply
- Wired for information technology/Internet access

Medications, medical records, and any medical equipment required by patients must be transferred, along with the patients themselves, during the transition to the alternative care site. To accomplish this, organizations might wish to consider developing a checklist to ensure that the patient has all of his or her vital information. It could include a medication list, a diagnosis or problem list, a medical history with the names and phone numbers of physicians, and a list of allergies and sensitivities. Organizations might also choose to develop an abbreviated medical record for use in a large-scale emergency that can be kept with the patients as they move through the system.

In addition, patients have to be tracked to, within, and from the alternative site. One of the best ways to ensure the accurate tracking of patients is to start with an accurate list of all patients and their locations within the organization. Some hospital associations are assisting members with this task by developing patient tracking systems. As part of the HICS, the Disaster Victim/Patient Tracking Form (*see* Figure 3-2, page 45) is an example of a tool that can be used to account for the location of patients receiving medical attention throughout a facility. The document has space to list the names, sex, dates of birth, triage area, disposition, and other essential information for up to 21

Be Prepared Tip

Choosing an Alternative Care Site

Develop a spreadsheet, placing factors from the list of items to consider when selecting an alternative care site on one axis and the list of potential alternative care sites on the other. Use a 0 to 5 rating scale (bad, poor, fair, good, excellent) for each factor to determine the best alternative site(s).

Table 3-4. Possible Alternative Care Sites

- Aircraft hangars
- Closed hospitals or nursing homes
- College dormitories
- Community/recreation centers
- Fairgrounds
- Government buildings
- Hotels/motels
- Libraries
- Meeting halls
- Military facilities
- National Guard armories
- Places of worship
- Schools
- Sports stadiums/facilities
- Tents
- Trailers
- Warehouses
- Unleased/empty open-space buildings (such as grocery stores)

Source: Joint Commission Resources: *Are You Prepared? Hospital Emergency Management Guidebook.* Oakbrook Terrace, IL: Joint Commission on Accreditation of Healthcare Organizations, 2006.

patients or victims of an identified event. It is designed to be completed hourly and at the end of each operational period, upon arrival of the first patient and until the disposition of the last.

Finally, patients and staff will require transport to the alternative care site. Ground transportation options include the following:

- Ambulances
- Ambulette services, which are equipped with wheelchair lifts
- Facility-owned buses or vans
- Family members' and volunteers' automobiles
- Prearranged use of local school bus company or school district buses

Inclement weather or poor terrain can make driving difficult; therefore, air transfer, such as helicopters, might have to be considered.

Figure 3-2. Patient Tracking Form

The effective use of designated incident management forms is another important part of incident management. The HICS includes 20 specific forms that are intended to assist hospitals in identifying the various types of information to record and archive during an incident. This is a patient location form used to track patients upon arrival and through disposition. All information must be meticulously entered and the form continuously updated.

HOSPITAL INCIDENT COMMAND SYSTEM

DISASTER VICTIM/PATIENT TRACKING FORM

1. INCIDENT NAME	2. DATE/TIME PREPARED	3. OPERATIONAL PERIOD DATE/TIME

4. TRIAGE AREAS (IMMEDIATE, DELAYED, EXPECTANT, MINOR, MORGUE)

MR #/ Triage #	Name	Sex	DOB/Age	Area Triaged To	Location/Time of Diagnostic Procedures (X-Ray, Angio, CT, etc)	Time sent to Surgery	Disposition (Home, Admit, Morgue, Transfer)	Time of Disposition

5. SUBMITTED BY	6. AREA ASSIGNED TO	7. DATE/TIME SUBMITTED

8. FACILITY NAME

PURPOSE: ACCOUNT FOR VICTIMS OF IDENTIFIED EVENT SEEKING MEDICAL ATTENTION. ORIGINATION: SITUATION UNIT LEADER.
COPIES TO: PATIENT REGISTRATION UNIT LEADER AND MEDICAL CARE BRANCH DIRECTOR.

HICS 254

Source: Reprinted from HICS IV "Hospital Incident Command Guidebook" ("Appendix D Materials – Forms"), Aug. 2006. California Emergency Medical Services Authority. Available online at http://www.emsa.cahwnet.gov./hics/forms.asp.

Coordinating with the Media

An emergency operations plan (EOP) should include policies and procedures for coordinating with the media, recognizing that emergency responses are improved when the media has been given accurate and current information. A 2007 study shows, though, that journalists and public health information officers (PIOs) often don't see eye to eye during disasters, with perspectives and organizational processes cited as limiting effective communication. Solutions to the challenge of sharing accurate and appropriate information include journalist participation in disaster exercises and drills, sharing of informational resources, and raising awareness at trade meetings.[1]

To the extent possible, the organization representative coordinating with the media should respond promptly and informatively to the media. The information must be accurate while also protecting patient confidentiality.

When speaking with the media, consider the following tips[2]:

- Speed is crucial in working with the media. Promptly call back reporters, as they frequently need the information to meet a deadline.
- Remain calm. If a reporter gets aggressive, stay focused on the question at hand and try to answer to the best of your ability.
- Never say, "No comment." It is okay to say, "I don't know."
- Look for opportunities in the interview to share key messages.
- Talk from the audience's or reader's point of view and avoid organization-specific jargon.
- Remember that anything you say during the course of the conversation could appear in print. There is no such thing as "off the record."
- If a reporter uses negative language, do not repeat it and do not repeat the question.
- Never argue with a news reporter about a story.
- Never flatly refuse to give information. Explain why the information is not available.
- Do not let a reporter put words in your mouth. Clarify comments when necessary.
- Repeating key messages is acceptable. Sometimes a reporter needs to hear a message several times and in several ways before he or she understands it.
- Answer questions directly, without giving more information than necessary.

References

1. Lowrey W., et al.: Effective media communication of disasters: Pressing problems and recommendations. *BMC Public Health* 7:1–8, Jun. 2007.
2. Joint Commission Resources: *Guide to Emergency Management Planning in Health Care.* Oakbrook Terrace, IL: Joint Commission on Accreditation of Healthcare Organizations, 2002.

Case Example: Pandemic Preparedness

Nobody has to tell you that health care organizations come in all sizes and offer all types care for all different kinds of patients. Let's look at how two vastly different organizations—a health care system and a small community hospital—are handling the planning process to prepare for a likely pandemic.

The Veterans Health Administration: The Nation's Largest Integrated Health Care System

Imagine providing medical, surgical, and rehabilitative care to 5.3 million patients at 154 medical centers and 1,300 sites of care, including 875 ambulatory care and community-based outpatient clinics, 136 nursing homes, 43 residential rehabilitation treatment programs, and 206 Veterans Centers.

That's the challenge faced by the Veterans Health Administration (VHA), the largest integrated health care system in the United States. In 2005 the Bush administration asked the VHA to come up with a strategy for dealing with pandemic flu. Although no one is certain about the exact biological characteristics of the next pandemic, it's likely to be caused by the H5N1 strain, known as avian flu. However, the VHA's plans and preparations must anticipate both likely and observed threats, such as H5N1, and threats from new, unrecognized strains of influenza virus.

"The number of people who are potentially eligible for our health care services is about a quarter of the nation's population, including veterans, their family members, and survivors of veterans," says Victoria J. Davey, R.N., M.P.H., deputy chief officer, Office of Public Health and Environmental Hazards, VHA.

Responding to the White House directive, the VHA named a 70-person team of staffers from all Department of Veterans Affairs (VA) divisions, including clinicians, hospital administrators, and infection control policy and leadership experts. These team members were divided up into work groups, and five months later, they delivered to the Homeland Security Council a 150-page detailed report on how to plan for and respond to a pandemic flu.

The plan is aimed at the VHA's stakeholders, including 25 million veterans, 235,000 VA employees, 93,000 volunteers, and 83,000 annual trainees. "We're also part of any federal report," says Davey, "so if an emergency is declared, we'd be working with civilian health care units and with health care units in other agencies, such as the Department of Defense. We're there for everyone who needs us."

A Model Plan

The Homeland Security Council rates the VHA's effort a "model plan," and other federal agencies have asked the VHA to share it with them. The plan explains how to prepare employees for a pandemic and how to handle space planning, infection control, supplies, heightened surveillance, staff illness, precautions for health care facility staff, mental health support for patients and staff, security, supplies, and many other subjects.

Another section includes instructions on responding to an actual pandemic, including information on refocusing patient care priorities, hand and respiratory hygiene, support for all ill staff members, antiviral drugs, vaccines, diagnostics, flexible work standards, recredentialing of the organization's retirees, changing demands and surge, advice line/telemedicine, fatality management, and security for health care sites. The final section of the plan deals with returning to normal operations and services following a pandemic.

(continued)

Case Example: Pandemic Preparedness, *continued*

"Health care organizations of any size will find the plan's 50-page toolkit section particularly interesting and useful," says Davey. "It features checklists for preparing for and responding to a pandemic. VA hospitals will use this framework to develop their own pandemic flu preparedness plans. They'll also appreciate the planning templates for use by local hospital management." The VHA plan is furnished in an editable format so hospitals can adapt different pieces of the plan to their own situations. "It will probably save them a great deal of time," says Davey.

So far, the VHA has distributed its plan only within the VA. However, after the mostly minor suggestions from the Homeland Security Council have been incorporated, the VHA pandemic flu plan will be available for download from the VHA Web site, at http://www.publichealth.va.gov/flu/pandemicflu.htm.

"Most of the questions we've gotten so far are about whether hospitals have to do their planning just the way we suggest," says Davey. "The answer is that we've tried to make this document very light on policy and instead offer suggestions that local health care organizations can adapt to their needs. Rather than, 'You must do this!' our tone has been, 'Consider including this.'"

Portrait of Northwest Community Hospital
Beds: 488 for inpatient and outpatient services
Inpatients per year: 28,500
Outpatient visits per year: 350,000
Physicians with offices throughout service area: nearly 1,000
Employees, including nurses, allied health professionals, and administrative and support personnel: 3,700

Northwest Community Healthcare: A Community-Sized System

Northwest Community Healthcare (NCH), which serves the suburbs northwest of Chicago, has been working on its pandemic flu plan since February 2005. The hospital solicited input from a broad multidisciplinary team within the hospital, including representatives from various clinical units, as well as from respiratory therapy, trauma, emergency medical services (EMS), the emergency department, radiation, oncology, infection control, and intensive care. NCH also held planning meetings with the regional Hospital Incident Command System.

The result of NCH's work is a four-page, tiered plan modeled on a plan issued by the Department of Health and Human Services. The plan explains what to do in case of varying levels of emergency, including a pandemic alert, seasonal influenza, a pandemic outside the United States, a pandemic inside the United States, and a local pandemic afflicting residents in the surrounding three-state area.

At each level, the plan deals with specific subjects, including hospital surveillance, hospital communication, staff education and training, triage, clinical evaluation and admission procedures, facility access, occupational health, use and administration of vaccines and antivirals, surge capacity, security, and mortuary issues.

"We've addressed as well as we can the unknown biological characteristics of a pandemic flu," says Mary Casey-Lockyer, R.N., C.C.R.N., the hospital's emergency response coordinator. "A plan like this can't be done overnight. Instead, we see

(continued)

Case Example: Pandemic Preparedness, *continued*

it as a living document on which we'll continue working for a long time. And we're partnering on it with regional, state, and federal authorities."

NCH is also planning regionally for alternative care sites for the minimally ill in case of a pandemic. "We're looking at which buildings could be used in case of a pandemic," says Casey-Lockyer. "We'll need clear criteria for hospital admission in case of a pandemic, and we're hoping that those criteria will be issued by our public health authorities at the county and regional level. We may have to ask our EMS providers to keep people at home and make sure they have fluids."

Respirators and Masks

One item that has proven controversial is the use of masks and respirators for staff members. Says Casey-Lockyer, "We are taking a risk-benefit approach by fit-testing a large percentage of our staff members, and we've alerted our N-95 vendors that we may ask them to fit-test some of our employees as well." NCH has stockpiled N-95 respirators and masks, and it's possible that the Illinois Department of Public Health would permit reuse of N-95s. "We have more than one per person, but no one can be sure how quickly these respirators would be used up."

NCH is considering a train-the-trainer approach in which it would train a corps of employees to fit-test other employees on a just-in-time basis. Casey-Lockyer anticipates that NCH might have some leeway on this in terms of time. "A pandemic in Asia would probably move fit-testing onto the front burner for us, especially since the World Health Organization is being so vigilant about tracking avian flu in various sites around the world as well as among our own animal and human population."

Communicating the Plan

The NCH home health care department presents guidelines on pandemic flu and emergency readiness at staff meetings, general meetings, and monthly emergency management committee meetings, and all this information is relayed to employees. In case of an emergency such as a flu pandemic, NCH would activate a pager alert system to its leaders, containing a dedicated emergency extension, which they would call to get instructions about whom to call back.

Partnering with Others

NCH is working with the EMS in the municipalities it serves. It also meets each month with the Northern Illinois Emergency Management Consortium, which has been coming together since the September 11 attacks to share concerns, plans, and information. During those meetings, NCH updates the participants on the medical and health aspects of various hazards.

"We've become partners," says Casey-Lockyer. "Hospitals are increasingly reaching out to the community and vice versa to plan for hazards such as a pandemic. That way, if I encounter trouble, I'll know that someone from a nearby community will lend a hand. Knowing everyone face to face reassures us that we all have each other's backs."

Source: Reprinted from Joint Commission Resources: Pandemic preparedness. *Environment of Care News* 10:5, May 2007.

Case Example: Long Term Care Organizations and Emergency Response

The World Trade Center and Pentagon attacks of September 11, 2001, showed the major role that long term care organizations could be asked to play during an emergency. Following the attacks, the Department of Health and Human Services (HHS) waived the three-day hospital stay requirement for Medicare coverage of nursing home care in the affected areas for the duration of the disaster. This allowed hospitals to discharge less than severely ill patients to long term care facilities. All long term care facilities in the area were required to report their bed availability to the HHS.

New York's Jewish Home and Hospital took a number of patients out of Lenox Hospital and Mount Sinai to free up the hospitals for the forecasted, but never materializing, deluge of patients. The long term care facility's own physicians and ambulances transported the transferring patients to the Jewish Home and Hospital so as not to call on the hospitals' ambulances and staff. The Jewish Home and Hospital also took a number of the more frail residents of Hallmark at Battery Park City, an independent and assisted living facility that had to evacuate all 75 residents and 40 staff members immediately following the attack. The evacuation went smoothly and nobody was hurt.

In addition, the New York Association of Homes and Services for the Aging, Jewish Home and Hospital, and other long term care organizations coordinated blood donation and other volunteer operations to assist the rescue effort. Long term care physicians and nurses volunteered their services in the triage areas set up at Chelsea Pier.

For Additional Assistance

- Hospital Incident Command System (HICS; through the California EMS Authority): http://www.emsa.ca.gov
- Center for HICS Education and Training: http://www.hicscenter.org
- U.S. Department of Health and Human Services, Centers for Disease Control and Prevention: *Long Term Care and Other Residential Facilities Pandemic Influenza Planning Checklist:* http://www.pandemicflu.gov/plan/LongTermCareChecklist.html
- The Joint Commission: *Standing Together: An Emergency Planning Guide for America's Communities:* http://www.jointcommission.org/PublicPolicy/
- American Health Care Association: *Disaster Planning Guide: A Resource Manual for Developing a Comprehensive Preparedness Plan:* http://www.ahca.org/news/nr060424b.htm
- Agency for Healthcare Research and Quality (AHRQ): *Emergency Preparedness Atlas: U.S. Nursing Home and Hospital Facilities:* http://www.ahrq.gov/prep/nursinghomes/atlas.htm
- AHRQ: *AHRQ Disaster Response Tools and Resources:* http://www.ahrq.gov/path/katrina.htm
- English J.F., et al.: *Bioterrorism Readiness Plan: A Template for Health Care Facilities:* http://www.cdc.gov/ncidod/dhqp/pdf/bt/13apr99APIC-CDCBioterrorism.PDF

References

1. Wood C.G.: Using quality to create a viable disaster plan. *Quality Progress* pp. 59–63, Jan. 1997.
2. Occupational Health and Safety Administration: *What Is an Incident Command System?* http://www.osha.gov/SLTC/etools/ics/what_is_ics.html (accessed Feb. 10, 2007).
3. Joint Commission Resources: Meeting the revised EM standards. *Environment of Care News* 10:9, Sep. 2007.
4. Hicks J.L., et al.: Health care facility and community strategies for patient care surge capacity. *Ann Emerg Med* 44(3):253–261, 2004.

Chapter 4

Establishing Emergency Communication Strategies

Cascading catastrophes such as Hurricane Katrina and the September 11, 2001, terrorist attacks underscore the need for effective communication during emergencies. Communication is fundamental to the business carried out by health care organizations on a day-to-day basis and becomes even more important during crisis situations. Effective communication both within the organization and with external agencies during an emergency helps to ensure the smooth implementation of emergency operations plans (EOPs).

The success or failure of an EOP is often determined by timely access to communication, ensuring the flow of critical information. More than just using the proper equipment, communication requires verbal and written interaction with staff and the community. This chapter, beginning with the Joint Commission requirements and expectations as detailed in Sidebar 4-1 (page 54), addresses the key components of communication during an emergency, one of the six critical areas of effective emergency management.

Emergency Communication Strategies

Though the standard focusing on reliable communications capability requires that organizations establish emergency communication strategies, the emphasis on communication as part of emergency management is not new with the creation of this standard. Rather, it broadens the requirements for effective communication to include ongoing communication with staff, the public, and the community. The standard also encourages organizations to strive for standardized communication both internally and externally. Although The Joint Commission does not require organizations to use the National Incident Management System (NIMS), some type of system like the NIMS is encouraged to ensure standardized communication across the organization and the community. (More information about the NIMS and other incident command systems is found in Chapter 3.)

In any health care organization, internal communication patterns develop and change to fit the day-to-day needs of administration, management, and care. Health care organizations also need to communicate externally with staff and private physicians; other health care organizations; medical testing laboratories; medical examiners; public safety services, including emergency medical services (EMS); and the general public seeking medical care or information.

The challenges associated with communication during an emergency are similar to other emergency management challenges—emergencies are by their very nature unpredictable and so are their effects on health care organizations and the communities they serve. In the event that community infrastructure is damaged and/or an organization's power or facilities experience debilitation, communication pathways, whether dependent on fiber-optic cables, electricity, satellite, or other conduits, are likely to fail. A mere forecast of an emergency also could in itself overwhelm vital communication services such as cellular phone service. Despite the barriers to communication during an emergency, organizations

Be Prepared Tip

Established Communications

Emergency communications procedures should be clearly defined, with an emphasis on coordination. These procedures should be a straightforward expansion of day-to-day procedures rather than a radical change in normal operating procedures.

Sidebar 4-1.

Applicable Emergency Management Standard

The organization establishes emergency communication strategies.

This standard requires the following:

- The organization plans for notifying staff when emergency response measures are initiated.
- The organization plans for ongoing communication of information and instructions to its staff once emergency response measures are initiated.
- The organization defines processes for notifying external authorities when emergency response measures are initiated.
- The organization plans for communicating with external authorities once emergency response measures are initiated.
- The organization plans for communicating with patients and their families during emergencies, including notification when patients are relocated to alternate care sites.
- The organization defines the circumstances and plans for communicating with the community and/or the media during emergencies.
- The organizations plans for communicating with purveyors of essential supplies, services, and equipment once emergency measures are initiated.
- The organizations plans for communicating in a timely manner with other health care organizations that together provide services to a contiguous geographic area (for example, among health care organizations serving a town or borough) regarding the following:
  - Essential elements of their command structures and control centers for emergency response
  - Names and roles of individuals in their command structures and command center telephone numbers
  - Resources and assets that potentially could be shared in an emergency response
  - Names of patients and deceased individuals brought to their organizations in accordance with applicable law and regulation, when requested
- The organization defines the circumstances and plans for communicating information about patients to third parties (such as other health care organizations, the state health department, the police, the Federal Bureau of Investigation).
- The organization plans for communicating with identified alternate care sites.
- The organization establishes backup communication systems and technologies for the activities identified above.

must plan for ways to overcome these obstacles in order to fulfill their responsibilities to patients, staff, and the community as a whole (as described in Sidebar 4-2, page 55).

Communicating with Staff and External Authorities

Clear and effective communication is critical in implementing the organization's EOP. In the absence of clear and credible information, health care staff, patients and their families, and the community as a whole can become increasingly stressed as speculation abounds.

Notifying and communicating with staff are important to successful emergency management activities. An organization's EOP should provide processes for notifying staff when emergency response efforts are initiated. Telephone, fax, and pager numbers should be noted and updated on a regular basis to be sure that necessary clinical, administrative, technical, and support staff can be reached initially and as the emergency progresses. For telephone numbers, the list should include office, home, and cell phone numbers. Knowing the best way to reach these individuals and maintaining a list of their next of kin helps to make this process go more smoothly.

Most organizations use a chain or pyramid format to communicate with staff in order to free valuable phone lines and staff resources necessary to carry out the EOP. Health care organizations also should consider having contingency plans to use radio or television stations to reach staff if telephone or cellular services are unavailable. For example, an organization's emergency management plan might include a process to notify the media whenever it is operating under special circumstances such as a winter storm warning or a flood warning.

Sidebar 4-2.

Communication Is Key

Communication is probably the most important of the six critical issues that can profoundly impact the outcomes of an emergency. Communication is so important because without effective, continuous, and consistent communication, all the other areas of emergency management would be unmanageable. Emergency response must be communicated and coordinated with staff, patients, families, and the community, including community responders such as police, fire, and emergency operations. Effective communication is critical to a coordinated response.

"The (pre-2008) emergency management standards require organizations to monitor communications during an emergency management drill. Organizations should expand upon that point and focus not just on monitoring communication but also planning for it," says John Fishbeck, associate director, Division of Standards and Survey Methods, The Joint Commission. Organizations should determine not only how they will communicate at the *beginning* of an emergency but how they will communicate *throughout* the emergency, given its changing dynamics. Also, the standard emphasizes the point that an organization should not just determine one method of communication to use during an emergency—such as walkie-talkies, cell phones, or satellite phones—but should prepare for backup methods of communication in case the primary method fails.

Source: Adapted from Joint Commission Resources: Preparing for a change in preparedness. *Environment of Care News* 10:5, May 2007.

Be Prepared Tip

Old-Fashioned Communication

In the age of instant communication through cellular phones, text messaging, and the Internet, it can be easy to overlook more old-fashioned methods for communicating. For example, having specific individuals designated to serve as messengers either within the organization or to the scene of an emergency, alternative care site, or community response center can ensure that critical information is relayed.

Staff members who hear the information would then call in for instructions about how and when to report to work.

Although some staff will come in spontaneously to lend assistance during an emergency, it is impossible to know how many will do so. Some staff might even be fearful of going to the organization if, for example, it has been involved in a bioterrorist incident or if there is a sense of lawlessness such as that seen in some parts of New Orleans after Hurricane Katrina.

For staff who are already at work, a public-address system can be used to make an organizationwide announcement that the EOP is going into effect. The announcement should also instruct designated on-duty staff to begin emergency preparations for their departments and to periodically report by a specified means to the organization's emergency management coordinator on the status of these preparations. A mobile paging system can be used to recall off-duty staff when the projected number of patients is expected to overwhelm on-duty staff. More information about staff roles and responsibilities can be found in Chapter 7.

Be Prepared Tip

Telephone Numbers

In addition to numbers for key staff, organizations should maintain a list of numbers of all of the departments in the organization, as well as pay phones and elevator phones.

Ongoing communication during an emergency is just as important as the original notification. If telephone lines and/or wireless communication are working after an emergency, the organization could have mechanisms in place to provide periodic updates, such as a prearranged telephone chain, or e-mail, voice mail, or fax messages. Written messages for staff could include using dry-erase boards set up at nursing stations throughout the facility or disseminating news bulletins. Organizations might also choose to set up several hotlines, including the following:

- One for family members looking for loved ones
- One for employees seeking information about the EOP activation
- One for medical personnel
- One for external authorities, vendors, or other stakeholders seeking updates

Having a protocol that details which mode of communication, including the various backup options, should be used during an emergency will eliminate confusion about how staff will receive emergency information. Not only should the communication modalities be predetermined, they should be interoperable and consistently used across the organization. Staff should be training to use the different types of communication equipment prior to an emergency.

The communications standard also addresses the need to communicate with external authorities in order to ensure a coordinated emergency management response. By notifying external authorities when emergency response measures are initiated and by planning for communication with external authorities, linkages can be put in place to manage and sustain operations. In other words, an organization's process for notifying external authorities of emergencies, including both internal and external events identified by the organization, is an important part of the EOP.

The incident commander should have a list that outlines the different types of organizations that must be contacted. The list might start with local entities, such as incident commanders at surrounding health care organizations, the fire department, police department, EMS, and the local health board. Next, the various local emergency management groups, such as the local emergency planning committee, county emergency operations center, community emergency response teams, citizens corps council, and/or area planning councils, could be notified. Organizations at the national level, such as the Centers for Disease Control and Prevention (CDC), the Environmental Protection Agency, and the National Guard, would be alerted next.

List of Key Internal Personnel

The incident commander should maintain an updated list of key staff members readily available in the event of an emergency. The list might include the following personnel:

- Hospital or long term care organization CEO
- Administrator on call
- Emergency department physician, chief (hospital)
- Administrative supervisor or house manager
- Director of security
- Chief nursing officer
- Director of engineering
- Director of infection control (hospital epidemiologist)
- Chief of microbiology/lab medical director
- Chief of medical staff
- Risk manager
- Public relations manager
- Information services/communications director
- Product resources director
- Director of pharmacy
- Chaplain/pastoral counselor
- Social services director
- Ethics officer

Source: Joint Commission Resources: *Are You Prepared? Hospital Emergency Management Guidebook.* Oakbrook Terrace, IL: Joint Commission on Accreditation of Healthcare Organizations, 2006.

For each entity, the list should contain an individual's name and instructions for how to contact him or her in an emergency. Consider mandating that key administrators, staff members, and marketing/communications personnel keep a copy of the emergency phone list at home and in their offices.

The CDC has devised a protocol for notifying local and state public health department leaders in the event of a bioterrorist incident. This tool can also be modified for use in the event of other types of emergencies. *See* Figure 4-1 (page 58).

Communicating with Patients, Families, and the Media

Dealing with people searching for their family members, with the media, and with those who do not need care but are worried can tie up scarce resources unless addressed as an integral component of emergency communication planning. Communication with

Staff Communication Difficulties

Communicating what is needed of staff can be difficult. First, the incident might not be recognized immediately as a large-scale emergency. For example, if the lights flicker and the hospital or long term care facility switches to emergency power, staff might wrongly assume that power has been restored to all areas. This is why it is important for an organization to have a way to inform staff that an emergency situation is occurring. Second, the organization might be operating on a "business as usual" plan when the internal emergency strikes. If the plan calls for staff to stop what they are doing and assume emergency-response tasks different from they are used to, the end result might be an uncoordinated response to the emergency situation. Staff need to know how to perform their daily routines to prevent an uncoordinated response.

the public during and following an emergency must be clear, credible, and consistent. This requires thorough planning in advance of any major occurrence. For example, organizations should think about issues such as the following:

- How do families and the community at large get news? Consider all of the available media outlets—radio, newspaper, television, and Internet-based options—and develop a list of contacts at each outlet.
- Are there any restrictions—either based on internal organization policies or applicable laws—on releasing information? Be sure to include these considerations in plans for emergency communication so that policies are followed even during emergencies.
- Is it possible to create templates for media advisories or news releases in advance? By using a fill-in-the-blank format, information can quickly be inserted and updated as conditions warrant, and the public can be kept informed.
- How will the release of information be coordinated with external agencies?
- Who will deliver information to the media and to the public? Designating a spokesperson—along with backups who can step in if the situation persists—allows the organization to communicate a consistent message.

One of the first steps to communicating with patients and their families under emergency conditions might be to establish a hotline that plays prerecorded messages that provide updates on the crisis while callers are placed on hold. Individuals staffing the organization's phone lines should receive training on relaying information to callers. By establishing a hotline that plays updated, prerecorded messages about the emergency and how the organization is handling the emergency, valuable resources can be directed elsewhere. A similar hotline can also be established for employees seeking information.

Be Prepared Tip

Communicating with Staff

Face-to-face communication with staff is an important part of responding to emergencies. To accomplish this type of communication, leaders can conduct personal rounds to all departments, provide standing-room-only briefing sessions, and hold routine update meetings with staff.

The prescripted messages could include self-care information for patients and descriptions of the steps the organization is taking to minimize risk to those being cared for at the facility. The messages could also explain the details of the emergency. For example, in the event of suspected anthrax contamination, the message could explain anthrax detection and treatment methods. This type of information could easily be obtained from organizations such as the CDC. Telephone operators should keep a list of phone numbers of other organizations to pass along to callers for further information. An example would be the toll-free Disaster Welfare Inquiry number of the American Red Cross, which can handle 50,000 phone calls per hour. When using information from external agencies or making referrals to external agencies, organizations should consider how to coordinate with these external agencies to deliver needed information to the public.

Organizations should also consider the need for fact sheets, brochures, and public service announcements to address the concerns of people who will physically go to the facility to obtain information. The same information can also be posted on the organization's Web site.

Figure 4-1. External Emergency Notification Procedures Recommended by the CDC

This page from the Centers for Disease Control and Prevention (CDC) Web site illustrates how the CDC instructs local and state public health department leaders to respond when informed of or suspecting a bioterrorist incident or threat.

What to Do in an Emergency >

Protocols: Interim Recommended Notification Procedures for Local and State Public Health Department Leaders in the Event of a Bioterrorist Incident

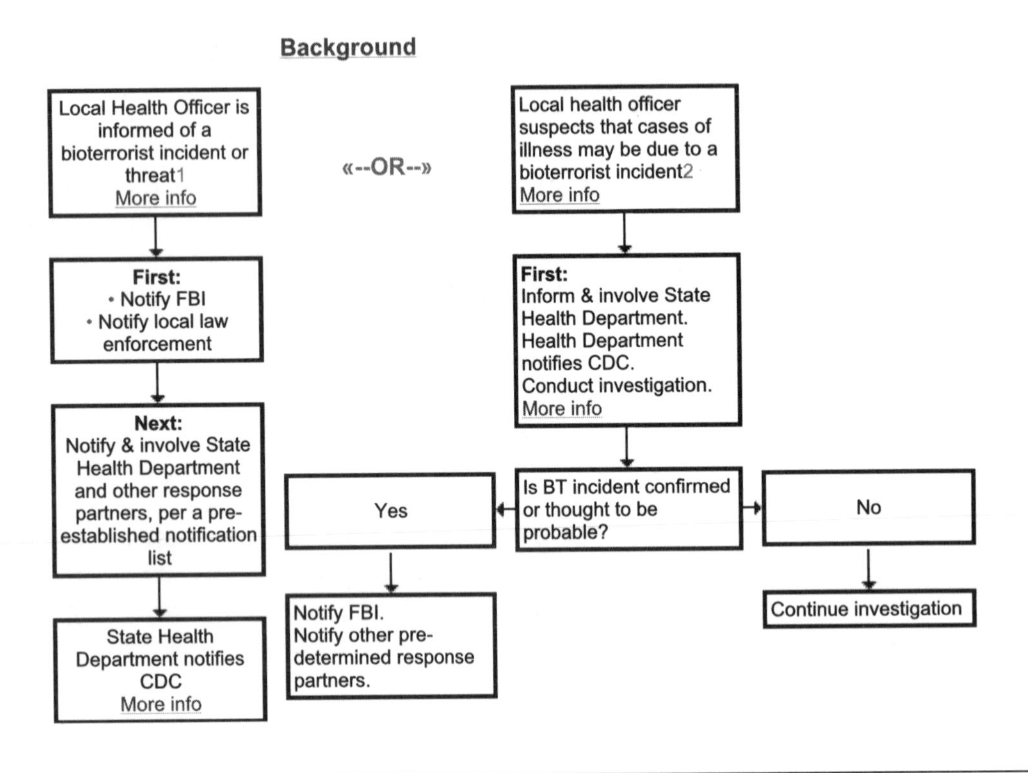

Source: Centers for Disease Control and Prevention. http://www.bt.cdc.gov/emcontact.Protocols.asp (accessed Feb. 22, 2007).

Organizations might also choose to create an on-site family information center in which pastoral care workers, social workers, case managers, and other personnel can provide information and support for family and friends waiting for information on the condition of disaster victims. Fact sheets addressing topics from how to cope with emergencies to symptoms of post-traumatic stress disorder can be distributed at the information center.

Other family and media communication planning issues to consider include the following[1]:

- Where will the public receive information regarding family members? Where will the media receive information regarding individuals receiving care in the facility?
- How will the public and media be directed to the area where information is provided?
- What information will be provided to family members? What information will be provided to the media?
- Who will provide information to family members? Who will provide information to the media?
- What provisions will be considered to effectively communicate with non-English-speaking individuals?

Sidebar 4-3.
One Country's Approach

Israel has an extensive structure for providing communication during an emergency that might be useful to study for ideas in establishing emergency communication strategies. Each Israeli hospital has an information center whose purpose is to provide reliable, accurate, and appropriate information during a national emergency. The center's functions include the following:

- Consolidating information regarding casualties admitted to the hospital
- Transmitting information regarding casualties to other information centers (regionally or locally) according to the need and situation
- Providing information to families
- Preparing family members for meetings with the injured person
- Providing psychological first aid to the family members of casualties
- Locating the family members of civilian casualties
- Providing information regarding unknown care recipients, including the collection of their photographs from different sites

The information center is staffed by the director of social services and includes a team of social workers, recorders, a computer expert, a physician, and security personnel. Signs direct people to the information center, which is located near the hospital entrance but is not adjacent to the casualty absorption area.

When a high-casualty incident occurs, the entrances to Israeli hospitals are closed off, to prevent the public from entering the care areas. "Consideration should be given to establishing a front information center to calm the public and conduct initial inquiries to identify relatives in the group and to regulate the public's entry to the main information center," notes the Israeli master plan. Personnel in the front information center locate the family members in the crowd and bring them into the hospital. Security forces help prevent people who have no need to enter the hospital area from entering it.

Information provided to family members by telephone from Israeli hospitals is limited to the fact that the family member is located at the hospital. No details are given about his or her condition until the family arrives at the hospital. Only a team consisting of a physician and a social worker provides notice to the family of a death. Information is conveyed to the media in Israel by the hospital spokesperson, the hospital director, or someone acting on his or her behalf.

Source: The *Israeli Master National Emergency Standard Operating Procedure for Hospitals* manual.

- What services will be offered to family members (for example, crisis/bereavement counseling, first aid)?
- What amenities will be offered to family members and the media (beverage/snack machines, public telephones, restrooms, and so forth)?
- What communications equipment is required?
- What staff are required?

Sidebar 4-3 (above) provides an example of the structure used in Israel to communicate with the public, family members, and the media.

Organizations should have a process in place for communication with news media, which can serve as a source of public education and community support. For example, the organization should consider designating a telephone line specifically for media requests and identify a spokesperson, such as an individual from the communications/marketing department (and an alternate for this person), to handle all media inquiries. If the designated spokesperson is a volunteer without any marketing or communications experience, then he or she should be given specific training on how to handle calls and inquiries from the media. A "news" or "advisory" page on an organization's Web site can also be used to offer information to the media.

Organizations should be prepared to provide information to the media on key topics such as the number of patients being received, the number of patients being treated, the types of injuries being treated, the number of patients that have been

BE PREPARED TIP

Establishing a Press Office

Maintaining or establishing a press office, staffed by designated individuals who know how to interact with the press and with local and regional health organizations, helps organizations be consistent in the information released.

released, and how patients that had been at the facility at the time of the emergency are being care for. In addition, organizations should identify a list of internal experts who can participate in press conferences and handle media questions. The contact information of these experts should be readily accessible. Other considerations include how to conduct regular press conferences, address rumors, and handle members of the media who come to the facility seeking information or an interview. Although updating the public with the latest information during an emergency is critical, it has to be done in a way that preserves patient safety and confidentiality per state and Health Insurance Portability and Accountability Act of 1996 (HIPAA) regulations.

Answering the following questions will help organizations manage media relations during an emergency[2]:

- Has an area within the organization been designated for receiving the media?
- Is the receiving area for the media located a sufficient distance from the emergency department or where patients are being treated, the command post, and waiting areas for relatives, family, and friends?
- Does the area designated for the media have telephone and television access?
- Has a staff member(s) been designated to control and take care of the needs of the media?
- Has a spokesperson for the organization been identified?
- Do staff know how to route calls or inquiries from reporters?
- Has the designated spokesperson been provided with a set of key messages approved by organization leadership?
- Has a plan been created to guide the internal spokesperson's communications with emergency management agencies or other lead community agencies?
- Are procedures in place for handling requests for information from the media and updating that information?
- Are procedures in place for responding to requests from reporters that are received after business hours?
- Are procedures in place for responding to a reporter(s) who arrives at the facility?
- Are plans in place for how the organization's Web site can be used to disseminate information and for how that information will be updated on the Web site?

Communicating with Suppliers

The standard under discussion includes a new requirement that recognizes the importance of communicating with purveyors of essential supplies, services, and equipment when emergency measures are initiated. This requirement ties in with other emergency management standards that deal with strategies for managing resources and assets during emergencies, but it primarily emphasizes the need for communicating with those individuals and organizations that provide the resources necessary for the organization to operate. The process used to carry out this requirement could be similar to that for notifying external authorities. For example, the organization should identify in advance those that provide essential supplies such as medications or linens, services that range from utilities to contract employees, and equipment such as personal protective equipment or generators. The health care organization should maintain a list of these organizations or individuals that must be contacted. The list could start with the supplies, services, and equipment most critical to the type of emergency situation at hand or to immediate operations and then move to those that need to be contacted as the emergency continues. For each purveyor, the list should include the organization, the name of an individual to be contacted, and instructions for how to contact him or her in an emergency. A copy of the phone list should be kept in a designated place in the institution, and organizations might also wish to consider mandating that key personnel responsible for emergency management keep a copy of this list at home and in their offices.

BE PREPARED TIP

Periodic Updates

Ongoing communication during an emergency is important to keeping internal and external constituents informed. Periodic updates can be delivered using methods such as a telephone chain, a voice mail system for recording messages for staff, or a mass fax or e-mail blast. Another consideration is the importance of coordinating with local and external agencies for accomplishing ongoing communication.

Seven Cardinal Rules of Risk Communication

1. Accept and involve the public as a partner. Your goal is to produce an informed public, not to defuse public concerns.
2. Plan carefully and evaluate your efforts. Different goals, audiences, and media require different actions.
3. Listen to the public's specific concerns. People often care more about trust, credibility, competence, fairness, and empathy than about statistics and details.
4. Be honest, frank, and open. Trust and credibility are difficult to obtain; once lost, they are almost impossible to regain.
5. Work with other credible sources. Conflicts and disagreements among organizations make communication with the public much more difficult.
6. Meet the needs of the media. The media are usually more interested in politics than risk, simplicity than complexity, danger than safety.
7. Speak clearly, with compassion. Never let your efforts prevent your acknowledging the tragedy of an illness, injury, or death.

Source: Covello V., Allen F.: *Seven Cardinal Rules of Risk Communication.* Washington, D.C.: U.S. Environmental Protection Agency, Office of Policy Analysis, 1988.

Communicating with Other Health Care Organizations

The Joint Commission's emergency management standards emphasize the fact that no organization can operate alone as a "silo" during an emergency. Emergencies that occur in one community can impact surrounding communities because of the potential needs for supplies, alternative care sites, and/or additional staff to treat victims.

Several of the elements of performance (EPs) under the communication standard address this aspect of emergency management by requiring organizations to plan for communicating in a timely manner with other health care organizations that together provide services to a contiguous geographic area such as a town, borough, county, or region. Specifically, organizations must communicate regarding the following:

- Essential elements of their command structures and control centers for emergency response
- Names and roles of individuals in their command structures and command center telephone numbers
- Resources and assets that potentially could be shared in an emergency response
- Names of patients and deceased individuals brought to the organization in accordance with applicable laws and regulations, when requested

These requirements have been part of accreditation standards prior to January 1, 2008, and are part of emergency management fundamentals that build capacity and identify resources that could be used during a crisis. Meeting these requirements will be made much easier if an organization has involved the community in its emergency management planning from the outset. As a starting point, consider the following leadership issues and questions for collaborating with proximate health care organizations:

- What health care organizations are geographically proximate (all types, whether offering similar services or not)?
- What proximate health care organizations offer similar services?
- What are the command structures of proximate health care organizations during an emergency?
- How will we communicate with proximate health care organizations?
- Who will be contacted at each organization?
- What similar resources (supplies, beds, staff, and so forth) might be shared or pooled in an emergency response?
- What might our organization be able to provide for proximate health care organizations?
- What might our organization need from each proximate health care organization?
- What in-kind or reciprocal agreements might we make with each organization?
- If patients must be evacuated from our organization, which neighboring organizations could receive transferred individuals?
- What supplies/vendors does each proximate organization rely on for materials that might be needed in an emergency?
- What backup plans do proximate organizations have for supplies in case of an emergency?
- How will information about the names of patients and deceased individuals brought to organizations be shared (per law and regulation)?

BE PREPARED TIP

Redundant Communications Encouraged

Provide redundant communication systems—cell phones, two-way radios, satellite phones, and so forth. Redundancy is a good idea because relying on only one system could leave an organization without communication options if the emergency knocks out that system.

When addressing these issues, it might make sense to begin with state hospital or nursing home associations for background information. For example, the Greater New York Hospital Association has compiled information about its members' emergency operations centers and key emergency personnel and capabilities.

Communicating with Alternative Care Sites

Communication capabilities with off-site facilities might be easier to address if, for example, the alternative care site is a government building, military facility, or a school. A closed health care facility, a tent, or a sports stadium, could pose more complex challenges. Regardless of where the alternative site is, organizations should consider how they will communicate about issues such as transportation, patient needs, staff, equipment, capacity, changing conditions, and other crucial information. In addition to traditional modes such as land-based telephones, faxes, and Internet access, organizations should consider more portable means such as two-way radios, cellular phones, satellite phones, wireless telephones, and so forth. Organizations might wish to develop a checklist to ensure that all communication issues are addressed.

Backup Communication Systems

When an emergency occurs, telephones and cell phones often fail and leave organizations without their usual means of communication. A contingency plan for backup of internal and external communication systems is crucial to ensuring that hospitals and long term care organizations can still communicate even in the face of the unexpected. Phone line options include maintaining a backup power source for internal phone switches, diversifying existing phone lines, and planning for the prioritized repair of existing phone lines. In addition, organizations should consider using satellite phones during emergencies, as these phones communicate using signals that are beamed to and from satellites, enabling them to continue to function when a natural disaster has damaged land lines or wireless telephone infrastructure. Table 4-1 (page 63) provides a list of communication equipment options.

Communications options aside from the telephone are the use of a public-address system and/or closed-circuit television system. Organizations might also use an alarm system that signifies when the facility is in an emergency-response mode. Any of these options could be followed up with messages on the organization's Web site and e-mails to all staff and employees.

Other methods for communication include wireless e-mail devices, such as personal digital assistants, 800 MHz radios, ham radios, and walkie-talkies. If possible, several radio transmitter/receivers should be equipped to operate on multiple frequencies, with dedicated channels in place.

The Radio Amateur Civil Emergency Service, which is regulated by the Federal Communications Commission, is a group of amateur radio operators who can be dispatched in times of emergency. Hospitals and long term care organizations might consider establishing contact with local ham radio operators who might be willing to volunteer their services during an emergency.

In addition, training appropriate staff to repair nonfunctioning communication equipment can help get the facility back on the communication track following an emergency. Because radio and microwave systems can be damaged, organizations should have available replacement supplies of antennas, coaxial cable, and other hardware that is susceptible to damage. Make sure that telephone lines coming into the communication center are buried, clearly marked, and protected from incurring possible damage.

BE PREPARED TIP

Telephone Line Locations

Keeping written records available for quick reference of telephone line locations will enable staff to easily locate broken equipment.

Table 4-1. Communications Equipment

Radio Equipment	Wire line	Combination
Two-way radio	Telephone	Cellular telephone
Pagers	Fax machine	Satellite telephone
Broadcast radio	Computer modem	
Television	Public-address system	
Satellite	Organization intercom	

Source: Joint Commission Resources: *Guide to Emergency Management Planning in Health Care.* Oakbrook Terrace, IL: Joint Commission on Accreditation of Healthcare Organizations, 2002.

Table 4-2. Communicating During Emergencies

Maintain an updated list of key staff members. Be sure to include the following personnel and their contact information:

- Chief executive officer
- Administrator on call
- Emergency department physician, chief (hospital)
- Administrative supervisor or house manager
- Director of security
- Chief nursing officer
- Director of engineering
- Director of infection control (hospital epidemiologist)
- Chief of microbiology/lab medical director
- Chief of medical staff
- Risk manager
- Public relations manager
- Information services/communications director
- Product resources director
- Director of pharmacy
- Chaplain/pastoral counselor
- Social services director
- Ethics officer

Identify a backup communication system. Organizations can use wireless e-mail devices, satellite phones, 800 MHz radios, ham radios, walkie-talkies, or a messenger system. Consider also creating plans to avoid overloading normal communication systems and maintaining the supplies needed to fix broken communication systems.

Notify external authorities of emergencies. Prepare a list of local and national authorities, as well as their contact information.

- Locally: Fire department, police department, emergency medical services, pharmacies, utility companies, essential vendors, blood banks, the local health board, city and county emergency operations center, community emergency response teams, citizen corps councils, and area planning councils
- Nationally: The Centers for Disease Control and Prevention, the Environmental Protection Agency, the National Guard, and the American Red Cross

Communicate with the news media. Identify a spokesperson as well as a list of experts who can participate in press conferences and handle media questions. Make sure staff members know where to route calls or other inquiries from reporters.

Communicate with patients and families. Establish a hotline specifically for patients and their families that can play prerecorded messages about the status of the crisis and what the organization is doing to reduce the risk of harm to patients.

Source: Joint Commission Resources: *Are You Prepared? Hospital Emergency Management Guidebook.* Oakbrook Terrace, IL: Joint Commission on Accreditation of Healthcare Organizations, 2006.

Yet another process that can be used to aid effective communication during emergencies and serve as a backup is a system used within the United Kingdom called Access Overload Control, whereby major mobile telephone companies reserve exclusive use of available channels for emergency services and local authorities at disaster scenes. This system allows calls to be made without being interrupted when radio/telephone networks are overloaded.

Table 4-2 (above) provides strategies for communicating during emergency situations.

Case Example: A Hospital's Emergency Response to the Virginia Tech Shooting

It promised to be a typical Monday morning at Montgomery Regional Hospital, a 146-bed general acute care and Level III trauma center located in Blacksburg, Virginia. A full complement of staff was scheduled to handle the day's variety of procedures. But early that morning, tragedy struck, and in a matter of hours, the day went from typical to unforgettable.

At approximately 7:30 A.M., two students were brought into the hospital after having been shot four miles away on the campus of Virginia Tech. One student was dead on arrival, and the other died shortly after. As the emergency department (ED) staff recovered from the shock of the first two shootings, a message came over the ED scanner notifying the hospital of an extensive, multiple-victim shooting at the university. Montgomery Regional Hospital jumped into action.

The following case example examines several aspects of how the organization coped with the emergency, including challenges related to communication.

Activating the Emergency Management Plan

"Our first step was to call a Code Green, our disaster code, over the public-address system to notify the staff there was an emergency," says Scott Hill, chief executive officer. "We also activated our call tree, which is used to call extra personnel into the facility." The hospital also activated its incident command system, as well as other aspects of its emergency management (EM) plan. Hill assumed his role as the incident commander, while Loressa Cole, chief nursing officer, immediately went to the ED and stepped into her role as operations commander.

Preparing for the Mass Influx of Patients

"At the time of the shootings, several patients were already in the ED," says Cole. "We quickly evaluated those patients to determine who we could discharge immediately and who needed to be moved out of the ED for treatment elsewhere in the hospital." Cole directed all nursing directors to report to the ED to help with discharging and relocating patients.

The hospital has a 25-bed ambulatory surgery department located adjacent to the ED. According to the hospital's EM plan, this unit can be used to treat trauma victims during an emergency. The hospital canceled all elective surgeries scheduled for that day in the unit and discharged patients waiting for surgery. "Within minutes, we had freed up our 16-bed ED and our 25-bed ambulatory surgery center, with the exception of a few patients who could not be discharged or moved elsewhere," says Cole. During this time, Cole also assessed the hospital's critical care department to determine the number of available beds for trauma victims as well as the status of the hospital's operating rooms (ORs). "Four ORs had surgeries under way, but they were able to complete within 30 minutes, freeing up not only the rooms but the surgical staff as well," says Cole. "Three general surgeons, one ear-nose-and-throat surgeon, and two orthopedic surgeons were available to assist in the emergency. As a result of the call tree, additional critical care and ED nursing staff came in, as well as several staff members who came of their own accord when they heard about the shooting on the news."

Before patients began arriving on site, the ED staff was in constant communication with the first responders to the scene. "The communication with the first responders was outstanding. Before a patient arrived on site, we knew he or she was coming, the level at which he or she was triaged, and his or her identified treatment needs," says Hill. That day, the hospital treated 15 more victims from Virginia Tech in addition to the original 2.

(continued)

Case Example: A Hospital's Emergency Response to the Virginia Tech Shooting, *continued*

Managing the Media

One particular aspect of security that proved challenging was managing the media. "Media were present from all over the world," says Charlie Smith, director of plan operations and security. "By locking down the facility and controlling access, we were able to contain the media in one designated area of our parking lot." Several Montgomery staff members were assigned to providing regular updates to the media, including issuing regular press releases.

Overcoming Challenges

One of the biggest challenges faced during the incident was communication. "Every director in the hospital uses a cell phone to communicate. Because of the nature of this incident and the need for students, police, families, and so forth to use their cell phones, the lines got bogged down, and it was difficult to maintain a connection," says Hill. "We are examining the possibility of using ham radios during future emergencies to prevent this issue from happening again."

The hospital also had to communicate in an efficient yet compassionate way with parents and family members of the victims. "Many parents called and arrived on site looking for their children," says Cole. "We quickly realized we needed a list of all the shooting incident patients at our site as well as those at nearby hospitals. By quickly referencing this list, I was able to tell a parent whether his or her child was being treated at a medical facility. If his or her child was not on the list, I referred the parents back to Virginia Tech for more information. Those were not easy conversations to have," he recalls. "But by having a process to follow, communication was streamlined, and we were able to provide as much information as we had at the time."

Working with the Community

Montgomery Regional was not the only hospital that treated victims that fateful day. Other area hospitals, including Carilion New River Valley Medical Center in Radford, Carilion Roanoke Memorial Hospital in Roanoke, and Lewis-Gale Medical Center in Salem, also treated victims. "Everyone really pulled together to respond to the incident," says Hill.

Montgomery Regional was prepared for a communitywide response. "We perform regional disaster planning, which includes all the region's hospitals, emergency medical technicians, police and fire departments, and even Virginia Tech's police department and rescue squad. Consequently, we had relationships in place before the event, which allowed us to have a coordinated and effective response," says Hill.

Addressing Security Issues

The emergency created several security issues that Montgomery Regional Hospital had to address. "Our organization typically has one security officer on duty during the day. After the first shooting, this officer came to the emergency department, locked down the department, and manned the area," says Smith. "After we heard about the multiple victims on the ED scanner, we activated the security portion of the EM plan, which calls for members of our maintenance department to back up security. With this backup in place, we had six more individuals responsible for security."

The hospital needed to quickly control access to and from the facility because of the large volume of media, parents, and friends of victims coming to the hospital. "We locked down the facility, including the doors. Only the main lobby door remained open. We also posted security personnel at each door to reroute people to the main lobby door, where identification was checked." The organization kept the facility locked down for seven days after the incident to ensure security for patients and staff.

(continued)

Case Example: A Hospital's Emergency Response to the Virginia Tech Shooting, *continued*

Addressing the Needs of Staff

"Shootings don't happen often in this town, and certainly not shootings of this magnitude," says Hill. "Even the first two shootings of the morning were traumatic for the staff, not to mention the entire incident." To provide immediate support for staff, the hospital relied on volunteer chaplains and other resources. The organization's contracted employee assistance program also provided counselors on site that day. "We made the counselors available to anyone who asked for help, including hospital staff, medics, patients, and friends and family members," says Hill.

Health care organizations across the country also reached out to help the staff at Montgomery Regional. "It was amazing the volume of e-mails, letters, phone calls, and flowers we received from individuals and organizations throughout the country, offering their support and encouragement," says Hill. "This outpouring of support also helped staff members cope with the event and its residual effects."

Lessons Learned

Although the hospital was effective in its response to the event, there are ways to improve. "We plan on doing an internal debriefing, as well as a regional one," says Hill. The governor of Virginia also called together a commission to further examine the event and how response efforts could be improved.

Source: Reprinted from Joint Commission Resources: Addressing a tragedy. *Environment of Care News* 10:8, Aug. 2007.

Case Example: Experiences with Emergency Communications

Hospitals participating in TOPOFF2—a large-scale bioterrorism drill led by the U.S. Department of Homeland Security in 2003 that simulated the detonation of a "dirty bomb" in Seattle and the release of a plague virus in Chicago—experienced several communication problems.[1] Among them were nonfunctioning walkie-talkies due to dead spots and unread e-mail messages from public health officials because staff were too busy "on the floor." Contingency plans included installing extra phones and new radio repeaters to cure dead spots, designating a staff person to monitor all incoming e-mail, and runners to carry messages to staff.

When the phones at Harborview Medical Center in Seattle failed due to being overburdened following an earthquake in 2001, administrators quickly addressed the problem. They broadcast a general page asking staff, employees, patients, and visitors to get off the phone unless they had an emergency reason, aside from the earthquake, for using it.[2] The 351-bed institution considered instituting a policy that when a Code Delta—the organization's disaster code—is called, nobody would be allowed to use the phone except for emergency hospital business, for at least 15 minutes. Afterward, department managers would designate one phone in the department for outside calls, and individuals would have to take turns using it.

Bellevue Hospital Center in New York City equipped its command post with 18 telephone lines, a computer, cable television, two-way radios, a copy machine, and a full staff, all of which played a role in maintaining both internal and external communications in the wake of September 11, 2001. Other communication tools used by city hospitals during and following the emergency included ham radios, combination call and two-way telephones, broadcast fax, and e-mail.

References

1. Rusting R.R.: Natural disasters: Responding to the unexpected. *J Healthc Prot Manage* 20(2):11–24, 2004.
2. Briggs S.M., Brinsfield K.H.: *Advanced Disaster Medical Response Manual for Providers.* Boston: Harvard Medical International Trauma & Disaster Institute, 2003, p. 35.

Source: Joint Commission Resources: *Are You Prepared? Hospital Emergency Management Guidebook.* Oakbrook Terrace, IL: Joint Commission on Accreditation of Healthcare Organizations, 2006, p. 62.

Case Example:
Homeland Security Exercise Shows Importance of Communication

In 2005 Hartford Hospital, located in Hartford, Connecticut, participated in the TOPOFF3 Full-Scale Exercise developed by the U.S. Department of Homeland Security to strengthen the nation's ability to prevent, prepare for, respond to, and recover from attacks involving weapons of mass destruction or from a natural catastrophe.

As part of the exercise, Hartford Hospital responded to a terrorist release of a chemical agent, testing its ability to manage casualties from this incident and its ability to plan and implement a recovery process. Hartford Hospital responded to the simulated attacks by activating internal emergency response plans, performing decontamination procedures, and collaborating in an emergency operations center to make necessary operational decisions.

After their organization's involvement in the exercise, Sandra C. Brown, bioterrorsim program manager in the hospital's Department of Trauma Emergency Medicine, and Dr. Lenworth Jacobs, director of trauma and emergency medicine offer the following communication-related advice to other organizations.

Good Communication Among Staff Members Is Essential

In exercises, as well as in actual emergencies, it is crucial that the hospital staff has effective means for communicating key information. For instance, it is important that enough radios are available for the security department and that there is interoperability of the means of communication when many different entities are collaborating on any event. Organizations need to have a plan for how their staff will communicate during an emergency and what the primary means of communication will be. If certain staff members in the field do not have access to a particular mode of communication, such as a Web site used to send messages to staff, the secondary mode of communication, such as radio contact, needs to be planned out in advance to ensure that all staff members can be reached.

Organizations should also ensure that their internal communications systems are adequate to deal with a large-scale emergency. It is important for caregivers who are triaging and decontaminating patients outside the organization to have a way to communicate with caregivers inside the organization. Hartford Hospital used a portable internal communications system for this purpose.

One of the means of communication used by Hartford Hospital during the exercise was satellite phones that were provided to all hospitals for this exercise by the state. These telephones, which served as a secondary mode of communication for the staff at Hartford Hospital, had the benefit of providing communications abilities to the hospital if the regular phone lines failed. Satellite phones should be used with guidelines that dictate how many organizations will use them at once, because they can be overloaded by too many organizations using them simultaneously.

Another insight from Hartford Hospital is that communication should be as precise as possible at all times. For instance, rather than asking the nursing unit if it can take 20 patients, it is more time-efficient to tell the unit how many patients are arriving so that it can prepare for them.

In addition, in a large hospital, it is important to have people on staff to serve as message runners. Having effective communication procedures between the emergency department and the pharmacy is also crucial during an emergency. It is important to know how to access medications and who can access the medications (including which staff members can serve as stand-ins to access medications when other staff members are not available).

(continued)

Case Example: Homeland Security Exercise Shows Importance of Communication, *continued*

Ensure that the public information officer has access to a medical expert. Although hospitals generally have spokespeople who provide information to the media, the public has a desire to hear from a medical expert. If such a person is available and ready to answer questions, he or she can be very helpful in assisting the public information officer in press briefings.

Source: Adapted from Joint Commission Resources: *Are You Prepared? Hospital Emergency Management Guidebook.* Oakbrook Terrace, IL: Joint Commission on Accreditation of Healthcare Organizations, 2006, pp. 142–146.

For Additional Assistance

Information about communications is available from a number of sources.
The Office of Public Affairs of the U.S. Department of Health and Human Services (HHS) and other HHS agencies have developed messages and other resources for use during a response to an emergency. For those new to communicating in a crisis, basic educational materials regarding crisis communication are also provided. Among the topics are the following:

- *Communicating in the First Hours*
- *Initial Communication with the Public During a Potential Terrorism Event*
- *Terrorism and Other Public Health Emergencies: a Reference Guide for Media*
- *Public Health Emergency Response: a Guide for Leaders and Responders*
- *Communicating in a Crisis: Risk Communications Guidelines for Public Officials*
- *Emergency Risk Communications*

The materials can be accessed at http://www.hhs.gov/disasters/press/newsroom/communication/index.html.

Organizations such as the American Red Cross, http://www.redcross.org, and the Federal Emergency Management Agency, http://www.fema.gov, also have emergency preparedness print advertisements, guides, educational materials, and fact sheets available that might be useful for communicating during an emergency.

References

1. Joint Commission Resources: *Guide to Emergency Management Planning in Health Care.* Oakbrook Terrace, IL: Joint Commission on Accreditation of Healthcare Organizations, 2002.
2. Joint Commission Resources: *Are You Prepared? Hospital Emergency Management Guidebook.* Oakbrook Terrace, IL: Joint Commission on Accreditation of Healthcare Organizations, 2006.

Chapter 5

Establishing Strategies for Managing Resources and Assets

In recent years, several large-scale disasters have resulted in less-than-ideal emergency responses. In some cases, resources ran out and patient safety was compromised.[1] To ensure an effective response to an emergency, organizations must consider what items will be needed to adequately care for patients.

In the event that an organization's community is affected by a disaster and cannot provide resources to the health care organization, plans must recognize the risk that some assets might not be available. One of the key things that The Joint Commission learned in studying the response of organizations to emergencies is that communities, including the health care organizations within those communities, cannot rely on the federal government in the aftermath of a disaster. Organizations should assume that they will not receive federal support and plan accordingly. If a large-scale event occurs, the federal government could be too stressed to provide the type and duration of support needed by an individual community.[1]

This chapter focuses on managing resources and assets—the second critical area of emergency response—and the importance of understanding the scope and availability of an organization's materials, supplies, services, and so forth. Sidebar 5-1 (page 72) details the Joint Commission's expectations related to managing resources and assets.

Assets and Resources During Emergencies

Organizations are required to develop strategies for managing resources and assets during emergencies, a concept that has been long been an integral component of emergency management standards. This standard recognizes the fact that organizations that continue to operate during emergencies must sustain essential resources, materials, and facilities in order to provide safe, effective care. The emergency operations plan (EOP) should identify how resources and assets will be solicited and acquired from a range of possible sources, such as vendors, neighboring health care providers, other community organizations, state affiliates, or a regional parent company. Emergencies that affect a broad geographic region or continue for an extended period, such as the circumstances seen during Hurricane Katrina, require planning. To address these possibilities, an organization's plan must proactively identify, locate, acquire, distribute, and account for critical resources and supplies. The plan should recognize that everything will not occur exactly as foreseen.

For example, multiple organizations might be vying for a limited supply from the same vendor. Or, vendors also might be affected by the emergency and have difficulty fulfilling their commitments. Because some assets might not be available from planned sources, contingency plans are crucial for critical supplies.

The infrastructure for supplying and supporting a health care organization is complex, but the hazard vulnerability analysis (HVA) will help identify risks to this infrastructure that can be mitigated. Planning must address managing and maintaining the facility, but also must consider evacuation of the entire facility when the environment is no longer deemed safe.

Obtaining and Replenishing Supplies

The issue of supplies is challenging in that organizations must plan for obtaining medical, pharmaceutical, and nonmedical supplies that will be needed to respond to an emergency, as well plan for replenishing those supplies. To address these issues, organizations can start by evaluating what supplies are necessary and evaluating what vendors are already in place. Keep in mind also that organizations must plan for self-sufficiency for an extended period of time—96 hours, as described in Chapter 3.

Sidebar 5-1.

Applicable Emergency Management Standard

The organization establishes strategies for managing resources and assets during emergencies.

This standard requires organizations to plan for the following:

- Obtaining supplies that will be required at the onset of emergency response (medical, pharmaceutical, and nonmedical)
- Replenishing medical supplies and equipment that will be required throughout response and recovery, including personal protective equipment where required
- Replenishing pharmaceutical supplies that will be required throughout response and recovery, including access to and distribution of caches (stockpiled by the organization or its affiliates, or local, state, or federal sources) to which the organization has access
- Replenishing nonmedical supplies that will be required throughout response and recovery (for example, food, linen, water, fuel for generators and transportation vehicles)
- Managing staff support activities (for example, housing, transportation, incident stress debriefing)
- Managing staff family support needs (for example, child care, elder care, communication)
- Potential sharing of resources and assets (for example, personnel, beds, transportation, linens, fuel, personal protective equipment, medical equipment and supplies) with other health care organizations within the community that could potentially be shared in an emergency response
- Potential sharing of resources and assets with health care organizations outside of the community in the event of a regional or prolonged disaster
- Evacuating (both horizontally and, when required by circumstance, vertically) when the environment cannot support care, treatment, and services
- Transporting patients, their medications and equipment, and staff to an alternative care site or sites when the environment cannot support care, treatment, and services
- Transporting patient information, including essential clinical and medication-related information, for patients to an alternative care site or sites when the environment cannot support care, treatment, and services

Be Prepared Tip

Surge Clause

Consider inserting a surge clause in contracts with prime vendors to ensure access to vital supplies. Organizations also might wish to prepare pre-emergency purchase orders that can be released to vendors, including out-of-state suppliers, during an emergency.[1] Finally, arrange for vendors to deliver extra supplies before any anticipated emergency events such as a hurricane, flood, or blizzard and return what is unused.

Reference

1. Pandemic purchasing priorities. *Healthcare Purchasing News* Jan. 2007. http://www.hpnonline.com/inside/2007-01/0701-PanedemicPurchase.html (accessed Sep. 19, 2007).

For small emergencies, materials already in the hospital or Medicare-/Medicaid-based long term care facility should be sufficient. A slowly developing incident generally provides the opportunity to order additional supplies. The organization must ensure that there is a store of supplies in case of an emergency and that there is a method for checking the cache on a routine basis.

The organization should also determine whether equipment will be needed by the local jurisdiction and should consider methods for getting some equipment to the scene of the emergency, if requested by the incident commander in the field. The request could be for expendable supplies, such as bandages and splints, or for items such as oxygen tanks, oximeters, and ventilators.

An emergency is also likely to create an influx of patients arriving at the health care organization. This will require that the organization have additional equipment, supplies, and staff to support the emergency response. Understanding the type of emergency and knowing the number of victims (as well as having planned for them in advance as part of the HVA) are important factors in managing resources and assets. Although organizations should have on hand supplies for the most likely emergencies as identified by the HVA, common additional supplies needed in an emergency situation include the following:

- Stretchers
- Intravenous supplies
- Oxygen
- Cardiac monitors
- Blankets
- Pharmaceuticals, including narcotics
- Orthopedic software and plastering materials

It is important to keep in mind the scope of activities that might be occurring in the community at any given time. For example, a fire at a large fertilizer plant might release a toxic substance that requires an antidote that is kept in only limited supply by the pharmacy. Realizing that the fertilizer plant is located in the community and that a fire is always a possibility, planning in advance for how the pharmacy would secure the needed medications will ensure an appropriate response.

Most organizations' HVAs include the possibility of an infectious disease outbreak and contamination. An assessment of the equipment and supplies on hand is an important component of planning for this possible emergency situation.

Be Prepared Tip

Knowing Your Neighbors

Know which suppliers and vendors other health care organizations in the community rely on for materials that might be needed during an emergency. Also, know what their backup plans are for supplies in case of an emergency.

Specifically, organizations should determine the current number of the following pieces of equipment: ventilators (adult, pediatric, neonate, and so forth), intravenous (IV) pumps, IV poles, suction machines, beds, stretchers, and wheelchairs. Then determine the current level of medical supplies, particularly items that provide personal protection, such as personal protective equipment (PPE), masks, gloves, eye protection, and face shields.

Organizations should make prearrangements with suppliers to receive hand-hygiene products, infection control products, and PPE in the event of an infectious outbreak. Organizations should also determine which vendors of durable medical equipment, such as ventilators, portable high-efficiency particulate air filtration units, and portable x-ray units, can provide these items on short notice. Because supplies might be limited, diverted, or sought by other health care organizations in the community in the event of a regional or prolonged disaster, organizations should also maintain a sufficient amount of these supplies at all times. Maintaining a list of key suppliers also makes sense.

Be Prepared Tip

Maintaining Supplies

On-duty staff who are responsible for finding and taking inventory of emergency supplies can use messengers, e-mail, fax machines, and so forth to send supply information to other departments. This effort should be coordinated and overseen by the incident command and the logistics officer. When disaster supplies are dispensed, a computer inventory of remaining supplies can be updated and sent to other departments by the same method. Also, supplies should be prepared to take to each identified care site for each triage category.

Be Prepared Tip

Supplies for Special Populations

When preparing the cache of emergency supplies, be sure to plan for pediatric casualties by having enough of the proper size of equipment or proper dosages of medications on hand or stored where they can be retrieved easily. Also, consider the needs of other vulnerable populations such as the elderly, disabled, or those with serious chronic conditions or addictions. (*See* Chapter 9 for more on managing clinical and support activities during emergencies.)

Staff Support Activities

Another important aspect of the EOP related to managing resources and assets is the inclusion of processes for managing staff support activities under emergency conditions. These activities include housing, transportation, and incident stress debriefing.

Housing is particularly important during an emergency because staff might be prevented from leaving the facility by inclement weather or other circumstances, which means that hospitals and long term care organizations might need to set up temporary shelter for staff. If housing does become necessary as the incident unfolds, organizations should have a predetermined area to house staff. Because staff members will need adequate rest and food, organizations also must ensure that there is enough food available on site. In the event that the organization runs out of food, it needs to have plans to obtain food, either from its usual food suppliers or from alternative suppliers.

Another issue health care organizations should plan for related to staffing involves staff's access to transportation or lack thereof during an emergency. When staff are unable to get to the facility because the roads are blocked, alternative transportation needs should be considered. For example, the organization might have to think beyond law enforcement, fire services, or other emergency response agencies, who are likely to be too busy with their own responsibilities to bring stranded staff members to work. Options to consider may be the National Guard or volunteer four-wheel drivers.

Staff might also require expert crisis counseling from behavioral health care professionals during and following an emergency. Organizations should consider having social workers, case managers, and/or pastoral workers available to conduct screenings to assess how staff are affected by the stress of the situation and to follow up with appropriate support. Incident stress debriefing helps staff process the emotions associated with an unusually stressful or traumatic incident. (*See* Chapter 7 for more information on the psychological impact of emergencies.)

During the emergency, providing information on a regular basis helps alleviate staff anxiety. Staff members need to have accurate knowledge of the situation, such as knowing exactly what has happened, how many patients to expect, and when to expect them, so they can prepare themselves and the facility for responding to the event. Keeping staff informed of the recovery process will keep morale high during what might seem like an arduous process.

Finally, staff support activities should take into account the needs of their families during emergency conditions. Like most people in an emergency situation, staff might be concerned about the safety of family members. Being torn between responsibilities as staff and as family members could add to the stress of working during an emergency. Among the questions to consider are the following:

- How will the organization handle the needs of staff members to contact their families?
- Does the staff have family emergency plans in place?
- How will the organization handle staff members who need or demand to leave to safeguard their own families?

Organizations can undertake a variety of actions to help staff manage their anxiety and to help them focus on the situation at hand. Organizations might consider setting up a call tree to help staff members communicate with their families in an efficient way that avoids overloading the phone system. Because people have a desire to be close to their families, particularly during times of crisis, organizations could set up temporary housing for family members or an on-site day care center if

Be Prepared Tip

Helping Families

In the event of a pandemic or a biological attack, an organization could serve as a distribution center through which staff members' families could receive vaccinations, antibiotics, or other necessary medications.

schools are temporarily closed. Although this standard requires organizations to manage staff family support needs, the examples of child care, elder care, and communication are simply examples; each organization should consider what types of support the families of staff members will require and how to properly allocate and manage those resources and supplies.

Sharing Resources

A new requirement of the emergency management standards is the potential sharing of resources and assets with health care organizations outside the community in the event of a regional or prolonged disaster. Sidebar 5-2 (page 76) offers recommendations for how to approach emergency situations in which organizations must help themselves rather than rely on government assistance.

Many organizations in the same region use the same vendors for the same supplies, whether it is linens, medications, or fuel. If the emergency is large enough to warrant hours or days of activities, with each organization relying on the same vendors to provide equipment and supplies, these vendors could exhaust their own inventories. Therefore, having a relationship with a vendor that is not in the organization's region is smart planning. Setting up credit lines before an emergency is much easier than trying to do so during the emergency. Some organizations might find it easier to negotiate with local or national health care associations to help develop shared vendor-purchasing agreements in emergencies. In addition, both health care organizations and vendors should have their own backups in place.

Evacuation-Related Issues

Although complete evacuation of a facility does not happen often, when it occurs as a result of a catastrophe, organizations must be prepared to efficiently carry out the process. Otherwise, the evacuation adds to the emergency and can itself put patients and staff at risk.

When the physical environment can no longer support care, the organization must have plans for both horizontal and vertical evacuation. Staff members must know their specific roles and responsibilities in preparing for building evacuation, know the location of equipment for evacuating or transporting patients, and understand how to carry out the actual evacuation. Issues to be managed during an evacuation include the transportation of patients, their medications and equipment, and staff. Organizations should consider whether medications will be provided by the sending or receiving organizations and keep in mind that some medications might be needed during transport. Organizations also should determine whether the

Resource-Sharing Questions

- What resources and assets (supplies, beds, staff, and so forth) might be shared in a regional or prolonged disaster?
- What could our organization provide?
- What might our organization need from other organizations?
- What provisions can we make to share or obtain resources and assets with health care organizations within our community during a prolonged emergency?
- What provisions can we make to share or obtain resources and assets with health care organizations outside our area during a prolonged emergency?

BE PREPARED TIP

Federal Evacuation Help

The National Disaster Medical System (NDMS), a federally coordinated system, is the primary federal program that supports the evacuation of patients in need of hospital care during natural or man-made disasters. Hurricane Katrina was the first emergency in which NDMS was used to evacuate a large number of people, and it brought to light problems related to evacuating patients from long term care organizations. Nursing home residents were part of the Katrina-related NDMS evacuation efforts; however, the program is not designed to serve this population because it does not have agreements with long term care organizations that could receive evacuated residents.[1]

Reference

1. United States Government Accountability Office (GAO): *Disaster Preparedness: Preliminary Observations on the Evacuation of Vulnerable Populations due to Hurricanes and Other Disasters. Statement of Cynthia Bascetta, Director, Health Care.* Washington, DC: GAO, May 2006.

Sidebar 5-2.
When Disaster Drives Cooperation

"In an emergency, local governments are likely to focus first on dousing fires, combating civil unrest, and evacuating homes and businesses," says Joe Cappiello, M.A., former vice president of Accreditation Field Operations, The Joint Commission. "Helping the local hospital is unlikely to be their top priority."

Cappiello points outs that hospitals that are part of a larger organization can count on receiving supplies, equipment, and support from their sister organizations outside the emergency area. But what about community hospitals and smaller health care facilities that are not part of a larger organization? These "orphan" organizations must plan on getting by on their own for several days following a disaster. In cases such as this, Cappiello has two recommendations.

First, he says, there must be more connectivity between the community and its health care infrastructure. "Each community must understand that its social fabric and its health care infrastructure are one and the same."

His second recommendation is for these smaller organizations to look beyond their immediate geographic area and begin advance planning with their suppliers and with other health care entities that have group purchasing abilities. "In case of disaster, the small organization will be able to turn to outside resources and depend on them to move supplies and equipment in their direction."

Source: Adapted from Joint Commission Resources: Pandemic preparedness. *Environment of Care News* 9:9, Sep. 2006.

Coordinating with the Media

Organizations seeking to ensure they have the proper assets and resources during an emergency should consider ways that the media can play a role in meeting that goal. For example, the media might be one of the only available communication routes during a large, regional emergency.

It is also important to remember that an evacuation of a health care organization is "news" and will require special consideration. The media can be a conduit for informing the public of an evacuation and providing information about the fact that an evacuation is taking place, why the evacuation is necessary, where patients are being transported, and how the organization has plans to ensure that patients receive necessary care. If an evacuation order is issued, organizations should also expect that members of the media will arrive at the organization being evacuated as well as at the alternative site. The public information officer identified in the incident command system should have plans for how to handle any such arrivals in order to provide accurate and current information while avoiding disruptions that could place patients, staff, or the media in harm's way.

original medical record or a copy should be sent with the evacuated patient, realizing that sending a copy might not be practical during an emergency situation. Organizations using electronic medical records or a combination of paper records and electronic records should also determine how they will address this issue during an emergency.

When developing evacuation plans it is important to consider the types of patients being relocated in order to ensure that the alternative site can meet the clinical needs of the patients received. This does not necessarily mean, for example, that a hospital could evacuate only to another hospital. It does mean that it would not be appropriate, for example, to relocate burn patients to a school gymnasium.

The emergency management standard relating to strategies for managing resources and assets also includes a requirement that organizations plan for the transportation of patients, medication, equipment, and staff as part of managing resources and assets during an evacuation. The transportation of patients was included in previous Joint Commission standards, but medication, equipment, and staff have been added to highlight the importance of these issues in providing safe, quality care during an emergency evacuation.

CASE EXAMPLE: A NURSING HOME'S RIDE FOR SUPPLIES

In the first hours after the September 11, 2001, attacks on the World Trade Center, the staff of St. Margaret's Home, a long term care organization located six blocks from Ground Zero, inventoried every department's supplies because they knew that there were not going to be normal deliveries the next day.[1] In fact, although the state Department of Public Health began sending supplies, St. Margaret's had trouble getting them. No vehicles were moving, and the supplies were being held up at the police checkpoints/incident command post. The organization's executive director rode his bicycle to the post to get the supplies released. In another instance, he rode his bicycle to meet the milk delivery truck and escort it back through police lines to his facility. The executive director faxed letters of entry for the vendors, giving the incident command post detailed information, including a physical description of the vendor.

Reference

1. Terrorism: Biological, chemical, nuclear readiness is imperative. *Environment of Care News* 4(6):1–3, 10, 2001.

CASE EXAMPLE: A HAWAIIAN HOSPITAL'S RESPONSE TO AN EARTHQUAKE

At 7:07 A.M. on Sunday, October 15, 2006, the ground began to shake violently on the Big Island of Hawaii. For the next 40 seconds, a 6.7-magnitude earthquake turned a peaceful morning upside down. Maryann Kaduk, the night supervisor at Kona Community Hospital, assessed the situation. She phoned the organization's CEO, Donald Lewis, at home to tell him that there was considerable damage to the hospital. Lewis is also regional CEO for the West Hawaii area of the Hawaii Health Systems (HHS) Corporation, which includes Kona Community Hospital—a 94-bed facility in Kealalekua, Hawaii.

Making the Decision to Evacuate

There were 69 patients in the hospital at the time the earthquake hit. The 40-second event rendered the hospital's long term care unit, medical/surgical unit, obstetrics (OB) department, and two of three operating rooms (ORs) unsafe for patient care. No patients or staff members were harmed during the earthquake; however, by the time Lewis arrived at the hospital, Kaduk had already made the decision to evacuate the previously mentioned areas based on their condition. "The evacuation went very smoothly, and no staff or patients were injured during the process. It is a testament to the skill, professionalism, and compassion of our staff that the provision of care was never interrupted," says Lewis. Kona's staff was well prepared for the evacuation procedure because the hospital has a disaster plan that covers potential evacuations and that is exercised twice a year.

Despite the damage to certain areas of the hospital, the intensive care unit (ICU) and emergency department were undamaged. "No one knew if we would be getting an influx of emergency patients from earthquake-generated destruction, so we kept those two departments open," says Lewis. In addition, the hospital's inpatient psychiatric unit suffered mild damage but did not have to be evacuated.

(continued)

Case Example: A Hawaiian Hospital's Response to an Earthquake, *continued*

Creating the Command Center

In accordance with the hospital's emergency management plan, the admitting department became the disaster control command center. From this location, Lewis was able to retrieve a two-way radio and contact Kaduk. The two conducted a brief walk-through of the entire facility. Parts of the suspended ceiling had come down, along with several light fixtures. Air-handling diffusers had been ripped apart, and toppled shelving was lying on the ground. The air was full of dust and dirt from the failing debris, and flooding from broken water pipes was occurring in several areas. Walls were cracked, and, in places, interior walls had separated from exterior walls. "The structural integrity of parts of the building became a concern, especially since possible aftershocks couldn't be ruled out," says Lewis.

After touring the hospital, Lewis and Kaduk returned to the command center and initiated the following actions:

- Activated the disaster recall protocol for staff
- Obtained a report on the status and disposition of all patients
- Set up a media response process
- Checked the status of the hospital's emergency water supply
- Checked the status of the hospital's emergency power supply
- Contacted the Big Island civil defense system and state emergency operations system
- Set up the hospital's patient emergency response system
- Determined how to contact the families of patients
- Contacted the HHS corporate office to apprise them of the situation

Moving Patients Outside

During the evacuation, patients were moved to several different areas. An OB patient in active labor was moved to the ICU, where she delivered a healthy baby later that day. The acute care patients from the medical/surgical unit were moved into a tent outside, and when that tent filled up, the organization moved patients under trees to take advantage of the shade. The hospital's 29 long term care residents were moved to shaded areas along the rear parking area of the hospital. Staff and supplies went with all the patients, and bedridden patients went outside in their beds. "While moving everyone outside to covered areas was an initial response, we knew we could not leave patients outside for too long," says Lewis. "The sun in Hawaii is very intense, and sunburn and dehydration were potential threats to patients' health and safety."

Finding Alternative Sites

The county civil defense plan identified a community meeting center as an evacuation site for the hospital's patients. "We found out in relatively short order that the earthquake had rendered that facility without power or air-conditioning, and there was no backup generator for the site. The center was not viable for patient and staff use," says Lewis. "We knew that moving people back into the hospital wasn't an option, so we had to come up with alternatives."

The administrative service building is right across the driveway from the main portion of the hospital, and it has two large classrooms on the lower level. After a quick assessment of the building, it was determined that although the upper level was damaged, the lower level was not and could accommodate the displaced patients. Hospital staff and civil defense volunteers moved classroom contents into nearby hallways and offices and cleaned the classrooms. All the medical/surgical patients—along with their beds, supplies, and staff—were moved to this location, where the hospital was able to provide care.

(continued)

Case Example: A Hawaiian Hospital's Response to an Earthquake, *continued*

By the end of the day, all patients who required continued hospitalization were flown to Hilo Medical Center, located on the east side of the Big Island of Hawaii. "We have an ongoing relationship with Hilo. Kona and Hilo are part of HHS Corporation's network of hospitals that exists throughout the Hawaiian Islands. We have standing protocols to help each other however we can," says Lewis. "Hilo is at least two hours away from Kona—if the traffic isn't bad and the roads are open; however, the earthquake made driving to Hilo out of the question," says Lewis.

Getting patients to Hilo Medical Center was a community effort. Ground transportation to the airport was provided by a local ambulance service. The coast guard provided a disaster medical assistance team along with a C-130 transport aircraft.

Kona's long term care patients were temporarily housed in the conference area of a local resort. "Our local fire chief had contacted the Sheraton Keahou resort, and they agreed to help," says Lewis. Spearheaded by the facilities director, the hospital moved the 29 residents, their beds, and other equipment—including a medication dispensing system—the nine miles to the Sheraton. Wheelchair-bound residents were moved in the hospital's handicapped-accessible van, and a local tour bus company made buses available to move the ambulatory residents. In addition, a local trucking company provided trucks and staff to help move the beds, tables, and other equipment the residents were going to need.

Establishing Relationships Before an Emergency

Prior to the earthquake, Kona Community Hospital had established a relationship with its community's emergency responders, including fire, police, county, and coast guard officials. One of the organization's annual emergency management drills is a coordinated drill with other community agencies. Through this drill, the hospital has become familiar with the capabilities of the community's disaster preparedness system. "We also have a dedicated emergency preparedness committee at the hospital, and the committee keeps abreast of countywide disaster readiness plans," says Lewis.

Managing the Press

Within one hour of the earthquake, the press descended on the hospital. Inquiries came by phone and in person, from all over the world. The hospital maintained a designated area for the press to congregate in the lobby. Via the command center, the hospital kept the acting public relations officer updated with minute-to-minute information on the status of the emergency response.

Ensuring Constant Communication

In the aftermath of any disaster, ongoing communication with all the key stakeholders is essential. To that end, Kona held senior staff meetings each morning, followed by a meeting with all department managers, which in turn was followed by a meeting with all available employees. A written status report summarizing key issues was produced daily and distributed to all employees, the medical staff, the press, and the corporate office. "Within several days of the earthquake, we did our first debriefing on what worked or didn't work in the emergency response. We wanted to get that information while it was still fresh in people's minds," says Lewis. "The feedback will be used to improve our emergency response system for the future."

Responding to the Emotional Needs of Staff

When dealing with the aftermath of a disaster, post-traumatic stress disorder should not be overlooked. Kona's medical director, who is also a psychiatrist, conducted postdisaster stress and anxiety counseling sessions for any hospital employ-

(continued)

Case Example: A Hawaiian Hospital's Response to an Earthquake, *continued*

ees who chose to attend. In addition, the local Adult Mental Health Division offered counselors to work with hospital employees. Both approaches helped employees cope with the psychological impact of the earthquake. "We are also fortunate to have healing touch and massage therapists associated with the hospital. We made their services available to our staff," says Lewis.

Cleaning Up and Moving In

Within hours of the earthquake, a civil defense structural engineer came to the hospital. He toured the building and told the organization that the building appeared to be structurally sound. Over the next hours, days, and weeks, the organization cleaned up and made repairs. Before moving anyone back into the hospital, all equipment and systems were checked and double-checked for safety and cleanliness as needed.

To acknowledge the efforts of staff, Lewis personally wrote to thank each employee and member of the medical staff. In addition, the hospital took out half-page ads in the local newspaper thanking everyone and every organization that came to its aid.

Source: Joint Commission Resources: Trouble in paradise. *Environment of Care News* 10:3, Mar. 2007.

For Additional Assistance

- Emergency Preparedness Resource Inventory, Agency for Healthcare Research and Quality: http://www.ahrq.gov/research/epri
- National Incident Management System Incident Resource Inventory System: http://www.fema.gov/emergency/nims/rm/iris.shtm
- Centers for Disease Control and Prevention, Strategic National Stockpile: http://www.bt.cdc.gov/stockpile/

Reference

1. Joint Commission Resources: Preparing for a change in preparedness. *Environment of Care News* 10(5):1–3, 2007.

Chapter 6

Establishing Strategies for Managing Safety and Security

The safety and security of patients is the prime responsibility of the organization during an emergency. As emergency situations develop and parameters of operability shift, organizations must continue to provide safe and secure environments for their patients and staff. Security is critical to enable the other components of an organization to operate in the way in which they are intended. Security staff must be present to ensure that staff can continue to carry out that plan, even if, for example, crowds begin to get agitated. They must also be prepared to protect the organization's staff and patients in the case of a disaster that results in a loss of social order, as occurred in the aftermath of Hurricane Katrina. In situations such as this, there might not be enough law enforcement personnel available to watch over the organization.

The third critical area of emergency management is discussed in this chapter and concentrates on a standard (as seen in Sidebar 6-1, below) focusing specifically on safety and security during emergencies.

Managing Safety and Security

Controlling the movement of individuals into, throughout, and out of the organization during an emergency is one of the most fundamental aspects of safety and security. The priorities of patient care and maintaining the facility cannot be accomplished without establishing internal security and safety operations. As part of emergency management planning, organizations must determine what types of security and safety issues are likely to arise. For example, organizations

Sidebar 6-1.

Applicable Emergency Management Standard

The organization establishes strategies for managing safety and security during emergencies.

This standard requires organizations to do the following:

- The organization establishes internal security and safety operations that will be required once emergency measures are initiated.
- The organization identifies the roles of community security agencies (police, sheriff, National Guard) and defines how the organization will coordinate security activities with these agencies.
- The organization identifies processes that will be required for managing hazardous materials and waste once emergency measures are initiated.
- Regarding hospitals and critical access hospitals only, the plan identifies means for radioactive, biological, and chemical isolation and decontamination.
- For long term care settings, the organization identifies residents who might be susceptible to wandering once emergency measures are initiated.
- The organization establishes processes for the following:
  - Controlling entrance into and out of the health care facility during emergencies
  - Controlling the movement of individuals within the health care facility during emergencies
  - Controlling traffic accessing the health care facility during emergencies

Security Planning

- Does the facility have the ability to lock down so that entry to and exit from all parts of the facility can be controlled?
- Have steps been taken to minimize and control points of access to and egress from buildings and areas without using lockdown procedures?
- Is a plan available to control vehicular traffic and pedestrians?
- Have arrangements been made to meet and escort responding emergency service personnel and vendors?
- Does the facility have the ability to communicate with individuals immediately outside the facility in the event lockdown is initiated?
- Does the plan designate how people will be identified within the hospital (for example, hospital staff, outside supporting medical personnel, news media, clergy, visitors)?
- Can staff gain access to the organization when called back on duty?
- Have provisions been made for internal traffic that allows patient movement through corridors and staff movement throughout their areas?
- Have egress routes for patients and staff been provided for evacuation purposes?
- Will elevators be staffed and controlled?
- Has elevator usage been prioritized (for example, casualties, supplies)?
- Have movement routes been designated within the organization and have traffic-flow charts been prepared and posted?
- Have arrangements been made for both vehicular and foot traffic to enter and exit the hospital premises?
- Have the following been established?
  - Uninterrupted flow of ambulances and other vehicles to casualty sorting areas or emergency department entrances
  - Access and egress control of authorized vehicles carrying supplies and equipment to a dock area
  - Authorized vehicle parking
  - Direction for authorized personnel and visitors to proper entrances
- Have arrangements been made for police support in maintaining order in the vicinity?
- Does the plan include a method to impact the management of vehicle and people convergence upon the hospital?

Source: Adapted from Association for Professionals in Infection Control and Epidemiology, Center for the Study of Bioterrorism and Emerging Infections: *Mass-Casualty Disaster Plan Checklist: A Template for Healthcare Facilities.* http://bioterrorism.slu.edu/bt/quick/disasterplan.pdf (accessed Mar. 10, 2008).

should make specific provisions for how and when the facility will be locked down when the emergency operations plan (EOP) is put into action. The bottom line is that security must be assured, or patients will not be able to receive the care that they require or staff might be unwilling to stay.

Coordinating with Security Agencies

In anticipating security issues, organizations should coordinate with the local community, such as the local police department, before the onset of an emergency. The health care organization should express its security concerns and identify the capabilities of community resources to support those concerns. For example, a hospital might assume that it can count on assistance from the local police department during an emergency. The police department might not, however, be able to offer any assistance or the level of assistance desired. Understanding what support is available will allow the organization to make more effective plans for security during an emergency.

In addition to the police department, this new requirement for coordination with community security agencies includes other groups, such as the sheriff's department and National Guard.

Organizations should also consider the need for collaboration with security agencies for other purposes. For example, travel access on roads or bridges could be restricted by security agencies during a disaster. Hospitals and Medicare-/Medicaid-based long term care facilities that identify the roles of community security agencies will better understand how to coordinate their own security measures, as well as how to allow for transportation of staff, patients, and essential supplies to and from the facility.

Managing Hazardous Materials/Waste

A new requirement in the emergency management standards is for organizations to identify the processes required for managing hazardous materials and waste when emergency measures are initiated. This requirement builds on existing environment of care standards related to managing hazardous materials and waste risks, recognizing that the special handling required of these materials and the need to minimize the risk of unsafe use and improper disposal are particularly important to consider during emergency conditions. For example, during an evacuation is not the time to begin thinking about what to do with chemicals, chemotherapy materials, radioactive materials, and medical wastes such as sharps, gases, and so forth. Or, if decontamination is required, how will the water be collected and disposed of?

Questions to consider might include the following:

- What types of hazardous materials and waste exist within the organization?
- What are the specific locations of these hazardous materials and waste?
- What are the normal procedures for securing these items?
- What are the normal procedures for disposing of these items?
- How will those processes need to vary in the event of an emergency (either internal or external)? For example, what if waste cannot be collected on schedule by waste handlers?
- What would the process be in the event of evacuation?

Isolation and Decontamination

Hospitals planning for security and safety during emergency situations must also consider radioactive, biological, and chemical isolation and decontamination. Contaminated patients must be segregated or isolated, and decontamination procedures to treat victims and protect other patients and staff must be quickly implemented.

An organization can take two broad approaches to isolation: The first is to outfit health care workers with personal protective equipment, effectively isolating the worker from the patient. The other approach is to isolate the patient from the worker. Hospitals and long term care organizations should conduct assessments, in advance, of current facilities and capabilities for airborne isolation. Organizations should evaluate whether rooms on certain units or even a nursing unit can be converted to negative pressure. Organizations should also evaluate mechanical and ventilation systems to support isolation and separation of air intake and exhaust in as many rooms as possible, if required. If the facility is planning any new construction, the ability to use some or all of the rooms for isolation should be considered.

Local Agency Coordination Issues

- What role will local law enforcement agencies play in assisting the organization during a communitywide incident?
- What role will local law enforcement agencies play in assisting the organization during any event—communitywide or otherwise—that exhausts the organization's security resources?
- How will the organization's incident command communicate with local agencies during a communitywide incident? What backup communication systems are in place?

Source: Joint Commission Resources: *Guide to Emergency Management Planning in Health Care.* Oakbrook Terrace, IL: Joint Commission on Accreditation of Healthcare Organizations, 2002.

BE PREPARED TIP

Security of Hazardous Materials

Ensure the security of biohazard and radioactive materials in the laboratory and elsewhere. Consider placing locks on all freezers and incubators that contain biohazard materials. Forward any suspicious inquiries regarding such materials to security personnel so that they can be in touch with external authorities as appropriate.

In the case of decontamination requirements, which are applicable only to hospitals and critical access hospitals, many hospitals have written into their EOP that the fire department will be responsible for decontaminating casualties. The challenge with this is that up to 85% of the victims of an incident involving hazardous materials show up at the hospital without having undergone any prior decontamination.[1] For example, in small incidents, such as agricultural or garage accidents, individuals will present themselves at the hospital emergency department (ED) without having called the fire department, and the hospital will need to perform appropriate decontamination. Because of this circumstance, hospitals should be prepared as part of their emergency management plans to assume responsibility for decontaminating these victims. Hospitals should continue, however, to coordinate with the community's local HAZMAT response team, which might have portable decontamination units and prefer to go directly to the site rather than risk spreading the contaminants to other sites, such as the hospital.[2]

Be Prepared Tip

Facility Security

Organizations should have a plan to secure the facility within a few minutes of an internal or known external biological or chemical incident in order to protect current patients, the facility, and staff. Entry should be permitted only to noncontaminated staff and decontaminated care recipients.[1]

Reference

1. *The Israeli Master National Emergency Standard Operating Procedure for Hospitals* manual.

The decontamination process involves isolating the contamination; decontaminating and treating patients; protecting staff, other patients, visitors, and the facility itself; and reestablishing normal service. The decontamination area should be a location with strictly controlled access. The best location for a decontamination area is outside the main facility because outdoor decontamination is preferable to protect staff, equipment, and other patients from becoming contaminated. Decontamination areas can be located inside the hospital as long as they have a direct entrance from the outside and a separate ventilation system that exhausts directly to the exterior of the building. Whatever type of decontamination facility is chosen, an organization should document its decontamination strategies in its EOP.

Preventing Wandering

For long term care facilities, a new component of the emergency management standards is the requirement to identify patients who might be susceptible to wandering when emergency measures are initiated. Because many nursing home residents have a loss of cognitive ability, it is essential to determine which patients will require help to prevent wandering during the chaotic atmosphere that typically accompanies an emergency. The risk for wandering increases when residents become upset or agitated or when they face stressful situations.[3] By identifying those individuals who might be prone to wandering, organizations can implement security precautions to keep these individuals in specific, safe locations during the emergency.

Controlling the Facility

An organization should determine the types of access and movement that will be allowed in the facility. This includes staff, patients, visitors, emergency volunteers, vendors, maintenance and repair workers, utility suppliers, and other individuals when emergency measures are initiated. Controlling access will likely include instituting a lockdown and then designating an entry point or points for staff and physicians, as well as for others who need access to the building. In hospitals, locating security staff in the ED to ensure that only authorized personnel can gain access is also important. If security staff are limited in numbers, organizations might wish to consider using fencing to block access to (but not egress from) certain parts of the facility.

Although the organization should have processes in place for limiting access to the facility to authorized personnel only, it is essential that those who are authorized are able to enter the facility quickly. To accomplish this, organizations should have procedures in place to identify care providers and other personnel during emergencies (*see* discussion in Chapter 7). This is important because if essential staff do not have some sort of identification, they might not be able to get through security roadblocks set up outside the organization.

One method to ensure that staff members can enter the facility could be to assign a security person to a check-in area outside any security perimeter that blocks access to the organization. That person would be given preprinted generic plastic badges and a list of staff and employees who are eligible for the badges.[3] Employees would be required to present picture iden-

Be Prepared Tip

Additional Security Staff

Organizations should have a contingency plan for hiring additional security staff as the normal number of on-duty security staff might be insufficient during an emergency. Options include contracting with private security officers or off-duty police officers. In addition, administrative and/or clinical staff could be assigned to provide a visible presence within the facility, such as at the entrances. All of this must be preplanned.

Be Prepared Tip

Crowd Control

If a crowd does form, the first step in gaining control is to establish a perimeter. Security personnel can also help to prevent crowds from forming by having clear information about how and where to direct patients and members of the community who might seek food or shelter from health care organizations during a disaster.

Coordinating with the Media

Several aspects of safety and security management are related to media planning considerations. For example, an event that requires isolation or decontamination of patients will be of interest to the media and to the community at large. By providing accurate, regularly updated information about the circumstances requiring isolation or decontamination, the organization can keep the public abreast of the situation. This will help to prevent rumors or speculation and will provide opportunities to inform the public about what, if anything, they need to do to stay safe and healthy.

Providing information about the situation as it unfolds could also be helpful in security issues such as crowd control. Supplying phones numbers to the public for information about their loved ones; preparing injury and casualty lists; and coordinating with the chaplaincy, social work departments, and the Red Cross on family notification can prevent large numbers of visitors from arriving at the facility and prevent those who do arrive at the facility from becoming agitated by a lack of information. This effort should be coordinated with community and state agencies and should be done to ensure that information provided is consistent regardless of which organization is providing the information.

tification so their name could be compared with the list. In addition, if an individual cannot physically be present at an entry point, video surveillance cameras can be used to monitor the access of individuals. Requiring personnel to wear photo identification, temporary badges, armbands, vests, or helmets could be helpful in distinguishing them from unauthorized individuals trying to gain access to restricted areas. Personnel might even be required to use swipe cards to gain access.

To prevent crowds from forming, organizations should have a system in place for organizing reporting stations, data collection points, traffic monitors, and waiting areas so that individuals can quickly be directed to the appropriate area. Organizations might even consider limiting visitors to only the immediate family.

For the individuals within the facility, organizations must consider how to control movement during emergencies. For example, organizations that have experienced structural damage would want to ensure that patients, visitors, or unauthorized staff, do not enter these potentially dangerous areas. Other situations, such as civil unrest, infectious outbreak, or biological attack, also demand similar considerations.

This process could involve a more localized method to limit access to the organization as a whole. For example, identification could be required not just at entrances, but at checkpoints within the organization. Or, electronic access control or other locking mechanisms might be used. Organizations should also post signs at various points in the facility to guide staff and other individuals. Sites for posting signs include exits on each floor, entrances and exits for each department, inside elevators, and so forth.

The final area that falls under security is traffic control. Ambulances, other emergency vehicles, and authorized nonemergency vehicles that provide supplies all must have unimpeded access to the organization. Consequently, the organization should have a plan to control access and egress of authorized emergency and nonemergency vehicles.

Case Example: A Lockdown Order During an Emergency

The Minnesota bridge collapse that occurred shortly after 6 P.M. on Wednesday, August 1, 2007, sent at least 50 vehicles and their occupants into a tangle of steel and asphalt that tumbled into the Mississippi River below. More than eight area hospitals were involved in the medical response to the disaster, including two Minneapolis medical centers that were particularly instrumental in providing care to the victims. Hennepin County Medical Center and the University of Minnesota Medical Center–Fairview, the closest in proximity to the site of the incident–to a great degree relied on their participation in emergency management exercises to adapt to the many challenges this tragedy presented.

Preparing for Multiple Emergencies

Joseph Clinton, M.D., Chief of Emergency Medicine at Hennepin County Medical Center was on his way to dinner with his wife at the time of the collapse. "I received a call from our on-duty emergency department (ED) physician who said, 'This looks like the real thing,'" recalls Clinton. "On my return to the hospital our team quickly began establishing emergency response procedures."

In this case, with Hennepin located less than a mile from the bridge, those procedures included sending a team of trained medical responders to the site to set up an incident command center. Working with other emergency personnel and even volunteers assisting in initial search and rescue efforts, Hennepin's team of physicians and paramedics provided care for the walking wounded and helped to direct the emergency transport of critical patients. "It was a chaotic scene, but in our [emergency management] exercises we have worked on bringing organizational structure to disastrous situations," says Clinton.

As a Level 1 trauma center, two to three times a year Hennepin participates in communitywide exercises of various types. "Our closest scenario to this event was a building collapse with 25 to 100 victims," says Clinton. "Like the bridge collapse, this was essentially a multiple emergency because we were dealing with many different types of injuries and with different elements that caused injury. Within the hospital and in cases where personnel respond on site, the key to managing an emergency is being prepared to make critical decisions. It's those exercises that equip you with the knowledge to make smart decisions."

This multiple-event approach to emergency management planning coincides with the Joint Commission's revised standards, which conclude that it is not sufficient to require organizations to plan for a single-emergency event; rather, they should be able to demonstrate sufficient flexibility to respond effectively to combinations of escalating events. The standards, which went into effect on January 1, 2008, emphasize a "scalable" approach that can help organizations manage the variety, intensity, and duration of disasters that can affect a single organization, multiple organizations, or the entire community. The standards describe specific operational requirements for health care organizations in planning a flexible response.

Adopting Flexible Emergency Practices

In the case of the University of Minnesota Medical Center–Fairview, the flexibility of its response evolved in the midst of a fluid situation and was reliant upon the Mock Trauma Team Activations it had recently coordinated. Donovan Taylor, R.N., Director of Trauma Service at Fairview, was headed home from the medical center when he received a call from the ED. A medical resident of Fairview in a high-rise above the bridge had called in to alert the organization to the unfolding emergency. Located just a block from the bridge, Fairview activated its Code Orange emergency operations plan (EOP), which included calling in additional staff and locking down the facility to limit patient access to a single entryway.

(continued)

Case Example: A Lockdown Order During an Emergency, *continued*

Unlike Hennepin County, Fairview is not a trauma center, but a transplant hospital. Its emergency staff, however, had spent the previous six weeks training and participating in Mock Trauma Team Activations as part of its ongoing preparation to become a Level II trauma center in 2009. "My new position is to help coordinate the pursuit of a Level II adult and pediatric trauma center," says Taylor. "Our exercises in the weeks before the incident included both adult and pediatric emergency scenarios with an unexpected number of trauma patients." the Joint Commission's standards require organizations to evaluate the performance of their EOP during planned exercises. "The (standards) also stress the importance of planning and testing response plans for emergencies during conditions when the local community cannot support the health care organization," says John Fishbeck, R.A., associate director, Division of Standards and Survey Methods, The Joint Commission.

As the core teaching hospital of the University of Minnesota Medical School, Fairview is made up of two campuses—its University campus on the east bank and its Riverside campus on the west bank of the Mississippi River. "It was our University campus on the east bank that received 25 patients from the collapse, while our west bank campus did not see any of its victims," says Taylor. Typically, trauma victims would be sent to Hennepin County Medical Center, which is also located on the west side of the river. "With the whole structure collapsing, responders had no way to get victims on the east bank across to Hennepin or our Riverside facility," says Taylor. Volunteers escorted some victims to the Fairview University campus. In one case, firemen commandeered a truck and drove victims to the medical center.

As victims arrived, some with spinal fractures and others with crushed lower extremities, Fairview's incident command post was notified that its initial lockdown order had not been accomplished. "Our information services (IS) and security dispatch are located in our Riverside campus," says Devin Mellors, emergency management specialist, Office of Clinical Affairs at Fairview. "We recognized that the lockdown had not gone through because the bridge collapse severed some of our communications lines with that campus. Through both radio and verbal commands, we quickly initiated an internal lockdown of the facility to ensure one access point."

With lockdown secured, Taylor recognized the need to bring the order and structure of a trauma unit to the frenzied atmosphere. Having honed his triage skills in the U.S. military, where he worked in the field with special operations units in the Middle East and elsewhere, Taylor and trauma surgeon Jeff Chipman, M.D., gathered staff in the midst of the crisis and began dividing them into teams. "We needed to be sure the expertise of our staff was evenly divided and focused on specific needs," says Taylor. The teams included at least one physician and two nurses, as well as members of ancillary departments such as lab and x-ray. Trauma teams provided care to the most severely injured, another team tended to those less severe, another was responsible for registering and accounting for new patients, and one team concentrated on existing patients at the medical center. "It all took only about 30 seconds to coordinate," says Taylor. "This team approach was just what we had worked on in our emergency trauma exercises, so staff members immediately assumed the roles they had practiced, and the emergency room quickly came under control."

Applying Insights from Emergency Experience

At Hennepin County Medical Center, similar measures were already in place. Despite its experience with trauma incidents and operations, its debriefing sessions with other local agencies and organizations continues to examine lessons learned—including the effectiveness of its communications systems during an emergency event.

(continued)

Case Example: A Lockdown Order During an Emergency, *continued*

"Fortunately, we were able to deal with the great volume of calls from civilians inquiring about the well-being of family and friends immediately after the collapse before redirecting those calls to a family reunification number operated by the Red Cross," says Mark Lappe, Director of Safety, Security, and Emergency Preparedness at Hennepin County. "Although our emergency radio lines and internal lines in the hospital remained open at all times, we are working with the Red Cross to more quickly establish a family reunification line in the case of an emergency."

As discussed in Chapter 4, Joint Commission emergency management standards now broaden the requirements for effective communication to include ongoing communication with staff, the public, and the community. "It also encourages organizations to strive for standardized communication both internally and externally," explains Fishbeck.

Since the bridge collapse, Fairview has dealt with its communications issues by adding a backup server and a duplicate security application on its University campus. "We have backup operators' consoles and 800 MHz radios on both campuses as well so that if we lose telephone lines we are able to communicate overhead," says Mellor. "Our debriefings on the emergency response have also been incorporated into our monthly Memoranda of Understanding meetings with 29 other hospitals in our area." Both Fairview and Hennepin County are working on Web-based systems that would more efficiently inform and direct staff that are outside of their facilities when an emergency occurs.

According to Taylor, Fairview's response to the bridge collapse highlights essential steps command and control should take upon learning of an emergency event, including performing the following actions:

- Implement the plan of care for current patients, establish teams for incoming patients, and lock down the facility in order to track new patients.
- In addition to the incident command, in the ED have a medical control person (an M.D.) and an operational control person (an R.N. with ED knowledge) coordinate care as quickly as possible while ensuring that they have necessary emergency resources such as equipment, medication, and an organized personnel response.

"The mindset here at Fairview is that it will happen again," says Taylor. "Even a car accident with four people injured can cause stress to an organization's operations." As the medical center continues to improve on programming aimed at gaining approval as a Level II trauma center, its staff has already gained insight and experience that will help chart their way forward.

Source: Reprinted from Joint Commission Resources: The Minnesota bridge collapse. *Environment of Care News* 10:12, Dec. 2007.

For Additional Assistance

Organizations seeking information on security issues related to bioterrorism, hazardous materials, and related topics can find references and resources online. These include the following:

- Institute for Biosecurity—Saint Louis University School of Public Health, http://bioterrorism.slu.edu/
- The Centers for Disease Control and Prevention, Public Health Emergency Preparedness and Response: http://www.bt.cdc.gov
- Johns Hopkins University School of Public Health and Medicine, Center for Civilian Biodefense Strategies: http://www.hopkins-biodefense.org
- The Environmental Protection Agency provides a four-hour decontamination program that can be offered without cost. For more information, visit the agency's Web site at http://www.epa.gov.
- The HazMat for Healthcare Web site, http://www.hazmatforhealthcare.org, offers four four-hour training modules for hospitals.

References

1. Briggs S.M., Brinsfield K.H.: *Advanced Disaster Medical Response: Manual for Providers.* Boston: Harvard Medical International Trauma & Disaster Institute, 2003, p. 35.
2. Joint Commission Resources: *Guide to Emergency Management Planning in Health Care.* Oakbrook Terrace, IL: Joint Commission on Accreditation of Healthcare Organizations, 2002, p. 49.
3. Joint Commission Resources: Emergency management in long term care, *Environment of Care News* 9(9):7, 2006.

Chapter 7

Defining and Managing Staff Roles and Responsibilities

When a disaster or emergency occurs, there is little or no time for staff training. It is also likely that staff responsibilities will change during an emergency. As new risks develop and conditions change, staff members will need to adapt their roles to meet new demands on their ability to care for patients. If staff members cannot anticipate how they might be called on to perform during an emergency, the likelihood increases that the organization will be unable to sustain itself during an emergency.

This chapter describes the importance of identifying the roles and responsibilities of staff members during an emergency. It also focuses on the need for organizations to inform licensed independent practitioners about what they need to do and whom to report to in an emergency. Sidebar 7-1 (below) details the Joint Commission's expectations related to defining and managing staff roles and responsibilities. This chapter also goes beyond the standards to explore the fact that the effects of an emergency are not limited to those who are injured by it, or even to those at the center of the emergency. During an emergency and its aftermath, staff in health care organizations experience significant disruption. Whether the emergency is intentional, unintentional, or natural, health care staff experience a wide range of emotions. No one who responds to a mass-casualty incident is untouched by it. Training as a caregiver does not provide immunity. It does motivate many to override stress and fatigue with dedication and commitment and to deny the need for rest and recovery time. This takes its toll on individuals and their families. To mitigate the psychological impact of emergencies on staff, organizations should consider the information and strategies contained within this chapter.

The Role of Staff in Emergencies

The emergency management standard discussed in this chapter describes the elements necessary to provide safe and effective patient care during an emergency. Specifically, staff roles must be well defined; staff must be oriented and trained in their assigned responsibilities; and staff must maintain their competencies over time. Staff roles in emergencies are determined largely by the priority emergencies defined in the hazard vulnerability analysis (HVA), and the reporting relationships in the command and control operations of the organization.

Sidebar 7-1.

Applicable Emergency Management Standard

The organization defines and manages staff roles and responsibilities.

This standard requires the following:

- Staff roles and responsibilities are defined in the emergency operations plan for all six critical areas (communication, resources and assets, safety and security, staff responsibilities, utilities management, and patient clinical support activities).
- Staff are trained for their assigned roles during emergencies.
- The organization communicates to licensed independent practitioners their roles in emergency response and to whom they report during an emergency.
- The organization establishes a process for identifying care providers and other personnel (such as identification cards, wrist bands, vests, hats, badges, computer printouts) assigned to particular areas during emergencies.

It is important to ensure that all staff members—including day-to-day staff across all departments and the medical staff—understand their roles in an emergency. Staff must be able and ready to adjust to changes in patient volume or acuity, work procedures or conditions, and response partners within and outside the organization. Organizations should document staff roles and responsibilities in the emergency operations plan (EOP), and can use a variety of formats—job action sheets, checklists, flowcharts, and so forth—to accomplish this task.

When addressing staffing issues in emergencies, organizations should consider the following strategies:

- **Define staff roles and responsibilities.** Consider how staff relate to the organizational capabilities and responses before, during, and after an emergency in the areas of communication, managing resources and assets, managing safety and security, managing utilities, and managing clinical activities.
- **Provide training for staff.** Staff educators, risk managers, clinical staff leaders, department managers and supervisors, or local authorities should educate relevant staff members on the organization's emergency management programs. Provide initial training and periodic refresher courses on areas such as hazard identification, triage, decontamination, infection control/isolation, treatment, and media and crowd control.
- **Create quick reference safety manuals.** Important emergency management information should be readily available in many places throughout the organization.
- **Identify and assign staff members to cover all essential staff functions under emergency conditions.** Determine in advance the availability of staff members on short notice, how quickly they can come to the organization, and how willing they are to work overtime. Include a protocol for alerting off-duty employees to come back to work.
- **Plan to provide adequate housing, food, transportation, and crisis counseling for the staff.** The needs of the families of staff also should be considered. (*See* Chapter 5 for additional information.)
- **Teach staff members how to manage stress.** Pass out information about coping with stress to all staff members, including how to recognize severe stress symptoms and signs of emotional stress and how to provide immediate psychological support to coworkers.

Be Prepared Tip

Who to Train

Organizations must decide who to train in emergency management. For example, which clinical staff (nurses, physicians, respiratory therapists) and nonclinical staff (administrators, security personnel, laboratory personnel) need training? Which departments should be covered? All staff, though, should understand that the organization has an emergency operations plan and know their role within that plan.

Staffing During Emergencies

Having policies that address the issues related to staffing outlined below enables organizations to have adequate numbers of staff members to respond to emergencies.

- How will adequate staffing during the emergency be ensured?
- Is a protocol in place to contact off-duty staff to report back to work?
- Is a policy in place to cancel scheduled vacations and days off during a disaster?
- Is a policy in place to deny vacations and days off during an emergency?
- Is a policy in place for extending staff shifts or requesting overtime?
- How are licensed independent practitioners included in staffing plans?
- Is the organization aware of state-specific laws and regulations regarding staff overtime or extended shifts?
- Does the organization have a contingency plan for staffing if personnel are either unable or unwilling to report to work?
- Is a plan in place to assist with the care of staff family members, when appropriate?

Source: Adapted from Joint Commission Resources: *Are You Prepared? Hospital Emergency Management Guidebook.* Oakbrook Terrace, IL: Joint Commission on Accreditation of Healthcare Organizations, 2006.

Defining Roles and Responsibilities

Staff members are crucial to the emergency management process, and this is a concept that organizations are accustomed to as part of emergency management standards. The standards are now more explicit, though, in that the organization needs to consider and plan for how staff fit in with each of the six critical areas of emergency management (communication, resources and assets, safety and security, staff responsibilities, utilities management, and patient clinical support activities). An organization's EOP should provide processes for identifying and assign-

More Personnel

At some point in an emergency, the situation will require more personnel, either to relieve those people who have been on duty for a long time or to supply additional resources to manage the emergency. Identify which personnel are needed to handle the situation. How will staff get to the hospital or long term care facility? Can they bring their families? Where do they stay if they need to spend a protracted amount of time at the organization? Studies have found that people in an emergency work best when they are performing familiar tasks or tasks they have specifically trained for.

Source: Adapted from Joint Commission on Accreditation of Healthcare Organizations (Joint Commision): *Emergency Preparedness in Health Care Organizations.* Oakbrook Terrace, IL, Joint Commission, 1996.

ing staff to cover essential staff functions and each of these six essential functions under emergency conditions.

To cover work shifts, the plan should determine, in advance, the availability of staff members on short notice, how quickly they are able to arrive at the organization, and how willing they are to work overtime. Plans should also specify where staff should report. Because an emergency might affect whether staff are willing or able to report to work, the plan should include a protocol for alerting off-duty employees of the possibility of being called for duty, canceling scheduled vacations and days off for key personnel, or denying vacations and days off until further notice. This might apply to all employees, not just key personnel, depending on the severity of the emergency's effect on the organization.

Most health care organizations struggle daily to maintain adequate staffing. Staffing during an emergency presents a particular challenge. Emergency management planners should consider keeping a roster of part-time employees, former employees, and recent retirees who can be trained in advance and summoned in an emergency. To do so, keep track of where former employees are working.

Staff Training

Orientation and education about potential emergencies and their expected risks and consequences, how to respond to each type of emergency, and how to provide the best possible care to disaster victims should be provided to health care staff before a disaster occurs.

This requirement (actually an element of performance) recognizes that staff education yields the highest "return on investment" in terms of resources expended versus improved response capabilities. An EOP should outline who is responsible for staff education at the hospital or long term care orga-nization. Although the nature and subject of the training will determine who leads the effort, administrators, risk managers, staff educators, or clinical staff leaders often assume responsibility for overseeing the education program. (*See* Table 7-1 on page 98.)

Because so many staff members require various levels of education—particularly in a complex hospital setting—department managers and supervisors might be best prepared to provide training in their respective areas. In fact, it is usually unreasonable to expect one individual to provide emergency management training for all new employees. Department managers and supervisors are typically best prepared to provide this orientation, with some oversight from organization leaders to coordinate the program and ensure completion of the program.

An organization typically will have a new employee orientation program that covers the broad environment-of-care processes and plans that apply to all staff, such as the fire plan and hazard communication plan. This is often based on the issues present in the department. Staff should receive initial training and then periodic refresher courses, though, because it is not enough to conduct such training during orientation alone.

Organizations must decide whether such education will be conducted on a quarterly, biannual, or annual basis. To keep the lessons fresh and in the forefront of everyone's minds, some organizations divide training topics into 12 modules that are presented on a monthly basis. No matter how often staff training is provided, it has to be repeated when staff turnover occurs, particularly if the individual leaving has a significant role in emergency management processes.

Formats for training vary almost as much as the individual roles and responsibilities during an emergency. Classroom or seminar settings can range from two-hour lectures to workshops that can last for several days. These can involve satellite broadcasts, videotaped programs, or live lectures. Many organizations employ a "train-the-trainer" model that involves

Staff Training Checklist

- Does the emergency operations plan specify responsibility for the training program?
- Does it include methods for unplanned training for new and altered roles?
- Does it provide ongoing disaster education material to facilitate staff awareness and currency of procedures?
- Does it have interorganization joint training sessions that deal with common aspects of disaster response?
- Does it track who received training and who still needs to be trained?
- Does the organization have ongoing, mandatory disaster training programs?
- Has the organization considered adapting disaster procedures for application when dealing with routine procedures so personnel can become familiar with them?

Source: Adapted from Association for Professionals in Infection Control and Epidemiology, Center for the Study of Bioterrorism and Emerging Infections: *Mass-Casualty Disaster Plan Checklist: A Template for Healthcare Facilities.* http://bioterrorism.slu.edu/bt/quick/disasterplan.pdf (accessed Mar. 10, 2008).

training a small group of employees who then train coworkers. Another format option is a self-study program, either computer or manual based, that staff can complete at home or in another setting.

"Just-in-time" training is often used as an adjunct to formal education sessions. This type of training makes concise knowledge available to providers at the time of an event and at the point of care. Many of the just-in-time educational components are Web based.

In-house instructors are not the only option for leading staff training sessions. Other individuals who might be involved include representatives of the state Occupational Safety and Health Administration office, local police or fire departments, emergency medical service or public health representatives, or equipment and pharmaceutical manufacturers.

Emergency management education, which can take place in the facility or off site, should not stop at the in-service level. Staff members must be involved in realistic exercises to test their knowledge. Being involved in disaster exercises enables staff to become more comfortable with, and more skilled at, engaging in emergency procedures. This, in turn, eases staff anxiety over emergency situations and improves their efficiency during actual events. A discussion of testing the EOP and staff-related components can be found in Chapter 10.

Organizations will want to consider staff training related to specific populations served by the organization. For example, a Medicare-/Medicaid-based long term care organization providing services to residents with Alzheimer's disease or a hospital with a large pediatric unit will want to train the staff responsible for implementing the EOP in how to effectively evacuate such individuals. Transporting confused elderly residents or frightened children requires sensitivity to the issues involved with their specific care needs. The effectiveness of educational efforts might be addressed through ongoing monitoring of staff knowledge and skills and level of staff participation.

BE PREPARED TIP

Verifying Compliance

To verify compliance with the requirements for staff orientation and education, The Joint Commission will not rely on sign-in sheets for the programs, nor on any other type of attendance records. These documents are important for other reasons, and must be maintained, but surveyors will instead talk with staff, usually during the building tour and tracer methodology process, to determine their knowledge of the emergency operations plan and the skills they need in order to fulfill their roles and responsibilities.

Staff members should be educated in the skills required to perform their roles within the organization's emergency management plan. Educate staff in at least the following areas described:

Hazard Identification

Every staff member should be trained to recognize possible hazardous situations and know how to appropriately respond to them. The type of training will, of course, depend on the staff member's role and responsibilities during an emergency. For example, clinical staff members should know how to identify victims who might have come in contact with biological or chemical agents. They should also know how to prevent a patient or resident from potentially contaminating the facility. Some staff members, particularly laboratory, pathology, or infection control staff, can be trained in epidemiological investigation. Security, reception, and administrative personnel should know how to react to a bomb threat. Self-protection from chemical or biological exposure, other toxins, and weapons must be specifically addressed and taught.

Triage

During an emergency, the objective of triage shifts from doing the greatest good for the individual to doing the greatest good for the greatest number of people. Therefore, the clinical staff should be educated in their organization's emergency triage protocol, which will differ from the usual triage protocol. Staff should know how to respond quickly and effectively to help a large influx of patients at one time.

Decontamination

The U.S. Occupational Safety and Health Administration mandates training for all staff involved in decontamination. In brief, First Responder Operations Level training is required for staff who would decontaminate victims or handle victims who have not yet been thoroughly decontaminated. This includes decontamination victim inspectors, clinicians who triage and/or stabilize victims prior to decontamination, security staff, setup crew, and patient tracking clerks. This level of training provides personnel with an understanding of how to recognize a potential hazardous materials problem and to respond accordingly. A briefing at the time of the incident, which provides instruction in donning appropriate personal protective equipment, information regarding the chemical hazards involved, and instructions on the duties that are to be performed, is required for staff members whose roles in the decontamination area could not be anticipated before the incident; for example, a medical specialist or a tradesperson, such as an electrician. First Responder Awareness Level training is required for emergency department (ED) clinicians, clerks, triage staff, and personnel who might identify unannounced contaminated victims and then notify the proper authority. This training is also required for security personnel, setup crew, and patient tracking clerks who are working near, but outside, a hospital decontamination zone. Some hazard communication training is recommended for ED staff and other employees who work in the ED but are not expected to encounter contaminated patients. Retraining must be provided on an annual basis.

BE PREPARED TIP

Centers for Disease Control and Prevention Guidelines

The Centers for Disease Control and Prevention provides guidelines that offer a framework for responding to various infectious disease outbreaks on its Web site at http://www.cdc.gov/ncidod/dhqp/gl_isolation.htm.

Infection Control/Isolation

Staff should be educated about the range of possible contamination, as well as the appropriate infection control precautions that should be taken when treated individuals with suspected or confirmed bioterrorism-related illnesses. These would include standard precautions and sometimes airborne or droplet precautions. Health care workers should also be trained in proper sanitation measures to contain the spread of infection.

Treatment

Staff members should be educated about treating illnesses and injuries they might not see on a regular basis or might have never seen. As a result of a terrorist attack, infectious diseases that were almost eradicated or are very rare, such as smallpox or the plague, could resurface. In addition, staff could be treating mass casualties or triaging an influx of infectious patients. Treatment protocols should be clear for all the aforementioned instances. In addition to treating the actual victims of an emergency, staff should be educated on how to provide this treatment without compromising the care of others in the organization.

The emergency management standards and other environment of care standards do not state a required frequency for ongoing staff education programs. Some regulatory agencies do have frequency requirements, and those must be followed. Often, other agencies require an annual retraining for compliance with their requirements. The Joint Commission is therefore

BE PREPARED TIP

Staff Assignments During Emergencies

When possible, staff should be assigned tasks that mirror what they ordinarily do at the organization. Studies have found that people in an emergency work best when they are performing familiar tasks or tasks for which they have been specifically trained.

not concerned with training frequencies unless they are specified in the health care organization's policies and procedures. The Joint Commission expects staff to possess the competence (defined as the knowledge, skills, ability, and behavior that a person possesses in order to perform tasks correctly and skillfully) to fulfill their functions in the environment of care. Annual training is certainly one way to accomplish this. As shown in Sidebar 7-2 (page 97) and Sidebar 7-3 (page 97), the issues of training for contract workers and competency-based education are two important issues to consider when addressing staff education needs.

Licensed Independent Practitioners

Licensed independent practitioners play a critical role in emergency management, making care decisions for those patients already in the organization and for those who arrive as a result of an emergency. It is therefore important that they understand their roles in emergency management in order to fulfill their responsibilities and meet organization needs.

The staff roles and responsibilities standard specifically requires organizations to communicate to licensed independent practitioners their roles in emergency response and to whom they report during an emergency. Organizations should work with their medical staff leadership to communicate expectations and outline roles and responsibilities of licensed independent practitioners during an emergency. The organization and medical staff should collaborate on this process as with other processes.

Identifying Care Providers

During an emergency situation, a health care organization might be dealing with a chaotic environment—damaged facilities, an influx of patients and visitors, extraordinary time pressures, and many other factors. These circumstances make it important to identify care providers and other personnel assigned to particular areas during emergencies. Organizations can meet this requirement in a variety of ways, such as by using identification cards, wrist bands, vests, hats, badges, or computer printouts.

Managing Stress

Because a disaster could be affecting the surrounding community, staff experience the emergency's immediate impact in much the same way as all other community members. They might or might not be able to get to work. They might or might not have lost their homes. Staff might have been injured or killed; their colleagues and families might be injured, missing, or dead.

To address the immediate impact of a disaster on staff, the organization's emergency management plan must address both of the following, as required by the standard described in Chapter 5:

- Staff support activities, such as housing, transportation, and incident stress debriefing
- Family support activities

Family support activities are likely to be of foremost and immediate concern to staff. Family support concerns include communication between staff and family and day care for children and adults. Leaders should consider how to facilitate the provision of both. They should also consider staff support issues related to housing and transportation. Organizations might also wish to address the issue of financial assistance. Staff might need financial assistance during the initial and ongoing phases of responding to a disaster. The organization should consider making provisions for this and offering convenience services such as check cashing so that staff members have easy access to cash. Sidebar 7-4 (page 98) details some of the concerns that impact the willingness of health care emergency workers to respond to a disaster.

Physical and Psychological Effects

Staff well-being is key to an effective emergency response and ongoing organizational effectiveness. Health care workers could experience shock, fear, grief, anger, and anxiety, as is common to other people involved in such an event. Their physical reactions could include tension, fatigue, edginess, difficulty sleeping, bodily aches or pains, startling easily, racing heartbeat, and nausea.[1] But they have the added stress associated with caring for victims during a time of crisis. Health care workers who respond to natural or man-made disasters are at high risk for secondary contamination, but an even higher risk for emotional distress.[2]

Rescue workers typically experience mild to moderate stress reactions during the crisis and in the early post-impact phases of a disaster. Some health care workers experience acute stress disorder, which is characterized by post-traumatic stress disorder symptoms that last anywhere from two days to one month following the trauma. It is estimated that as many as one out of every three rescue workers experience severe stress symptoms.[1]

Other longer-term psychological problems that can result from exposure to disasters include alcohol or substance abuse, anxiety, somatization, domestic violence, and difficulties in daily functioning. Another condition that can result from health care work-

Sidebar 7-2.
Training Contract Workers

Organizations often raise questions about required orientation and education for contract workers—individuals who work in the health care organization's building but who are employed by another entity. Examples of contract workers include agency nurses, contract tradespeople, or medical equipment service organization employees. The Joint Commission views these individuals as the contracting organization's employees, and, therefore, they must undergo some sort of orientation and education process.

Remembering that the training is role-specific (one size does not fit all), the contract staff does not have to undergo the same orientation and education as regular staff employees. The training does not even have to be done by someone in the organization; often the contract includes language stating that the contractor is responsible for orientation and education to the organization's specifications. Still, the health care organization ultimately holds the responsibility, and someone in the organization must ensure that the emergency management and other required training occurs.

Sidebar 7-3.
Emergency Preparedness and Staff Competency

Competency-based education for emergency preparedness is a relatively recent development in health care. One approach is to employ seven "cross-cutting" competencies that address the following[1]:

- Recognize a potential critical event and implement initial actions.
- Apply the principles of critical event management.
- Demonstrate critical event safety principles.
- Understand the institutional emergency operations plan.
- Demonstrate effective critical event communications.
- Understand the incident command system and your role in it.
- Demonstrate the knowledge and skills needed to fulfill your role during a critical event.

An approach to core competencies specific to nurses includes the following[2]:

- Describe the organization's role in responding to a range of emergencies that might arise.
- Describe the chain of command in emergency response.
- Identify and locate the organization's emergency response plan (or the pertinent portion of it).
- Describe emergency response functions or roles and demonstrate them in regularly performed drills.
- Demonstrate the use of equipment (including personal protective equipment) and the skills required in emergency response during regular drills.
- Demonstrate the correct operation of all equipment used for emergency communication.
- Identify the limits of your own knowledge, skills, and authority, and identify key system resources for referring matters that exceed these limits.
- Apply creative problem-solving skills and flexible thinking to the situation, within the confines of your role, and evaluate the effectiveness of all actions taken.
- Recognize deviations from the norm that might indicate an emergency and describe appropriate action.
- Participate in continuing education to maintain up-to-date knowledge in relevant areas.
- Participate in evaluating every drill or response and identify necessary changes to the plan.

References

1. Hsu E.B., et al.: Healthcare worker competencies for disaster training. *BMC Med Educ* 6(19):1–8, 2006.
2. Gebbie K.M., Qureshi K.: Emergency and disaster preparedness: Core competencies for nurses. *Am J Nurs* 102(1):46–51, 2002.

Table 7-1. Training for Disasters

When a disaster plan is in place, staff must be trained in how to respond to a disaster situation. An Agency for Healthcare Research and Quality review of current research found that training should include a combination of the following:

- Traditional educational methods, including lectures, discussions, audiovisuals, and written materials
- Teleconferencing, which can reach a large audience
- "Smart" patients or mock victims, which are helpful for one-on-one training but less practical for training large numbers
- Theoretical, "paper" drills, which do not require physical movement of patients, personnel, or equipment but usually focus on the roles and responsibilities and system integration components
- Computer simulations, which can potentially replace expensive drills and identify weaknesses in disaster planning
- Physical drills, which can improve knowledge of the disaster plan and highlight weaknesses

Source: Agency for Healthcare Research and Quality (AHRQ): *Bioterrorism and Health System Preparedness: Disaster Planning Drills and Readiness Assessment.* Rockville, MD: AHRQ, Jan. 2004.

Sidebar 7-4.

Willingness to Respond

Although many health care emergency workers are quite selfless in their efforts to care for others, their own personal safety as well as that of their families will also be on their minds during a disaster, particularly during a large-scale event.

One study found that emergency medical technicians were far more willing to respond to disasters in which they were at less personal risk, such as in a large fire with a high number of victims, than in a smallpox outbreak or bioterrorism incident. This information could reflect a response to the number of rescue workers who were killed in the September 11, 2001, attacks on the World Trade Center. Sense of responsibility (83.3%) and ability to provide care (77.3%) were most commonly given as the reasons by those who said they would be willing to respond; concern for family (44.4%) was the most common reason respondents said that they would not be willing to respond. (*See* Chapter 5 for more information about support activities to meet the needs of staff and their families.)

Source: DiMaggio C., et al.: The willingness of U.S. emergency medical technicians to respond to terrorist incidents. *Biosecur Bioterror* 3:331–337, 2005.

ers responding to an emergency is known as critical incident stress.[3] Symptoms include deterioration in one's sense of well-being, exhaustion, depression, hostility, lost tolerance for victims, dread of new encounters, guilt, helplessness, or isolation. This syndrome lowers group morale, increases absenteeism, interferes with mutual support, and adversely affects home life.

Staying Healthy

Disaster and response workers face unique stressors, which is why it is so important for health care organizations to educate staff on how to manage the stress that will naturally arise in an emergency situation. Strategies to manage stress during an emergency that can be passed on to staff members include the following[4]:

- Developing a "buddy" system so that staff members can monitor one another's stress levels
- Encouraging and supporting their coworkers
- Limiting shifts to no more than 12 hours per day
- Taking a break when they feel their stamina, coordination, or tolerance for irritation is diminishing
- Defusing briefly when they experience troubling incidents and after each work shift
- Making work rotations from high-stress to lower-stress functions and from the scene to routine assignments, as possible
- Talking about their emotions to process what they have seen and done
- Using available counseling assistance programs
- Participating in memorials, rituals, and use of symbols as a means to express feelings
- Taking care of themselves by eating small quantities of food and drinking water frequently
- Staying in touch with family and friends

Sidebar 7-5.

Leadership Strategies

Leaders can use the following strategies, provided by the National Mental Health Association, after an emergency to help their workforce cope and continue to work effectively[1]:

- Speak to the entire organizations as soon as possible. Leaders should meet with staff at all levels to express shared grief, as well as to promote available counseling services and other resources. Encouraging employees to take care of themselves is also important.
- Educate supervisors and managers. It is important for supervisors and managers to recognize the signs of emotional distress and to know about available treatment resources; encourage them or their staff to seek treatment when necessary.
- Provide educational resources for treatment resources.
- Facilitate communication among employees. Support among colleagues can help employees work through difficulties.
- Consider bringing a professional counselor/facilitator on site. Group meetings and individual counseling can identify those who need help and ensure that they receive the help, thus reducing the need for services down the road.
- Revamp your leave policy temporarily. Allow people time off beyond the norm for donating blood, community activity, and personal needs. Employees will benefit from feeling that they are able to take positive action and make a difference.
- Let business resume. Returning to productive work, while acknowledging that things have changed, will help with individual and organizational healing.
- Reconsider current travel needs. Consider postponing or canceling conferences or other meetings that require travel, recognizing that recent events might make people hesitant to make business trips for some time.
- Hold a memorial service. Such a service can honor the losses of employees' loved ones, as well as all the victims.
- Organize community action. Holding a blood drive, starting a voluntary collection fund for relief efforts, or similar actions demonstrate to employees that the organization is committed to helping those both within and outside the organization.
- Plan for future emergencies. Review the emergency operations plan to address any problems that arose with the recent disaster, and make sure to involve all segments of the staff in the planning.

Reference

1. National Mental Health Association: *Helping Your Workforce Cope and Return to Work.* http://www1.nmha.org/reassurance/workforce.cfm (accessed Nov. 16, 2007).

The need for immediate expert crisis counseling and spiritual support for all staff during a disaster should not be underestimated. Organizations should arrange for a skilled team of counselors and pastoral workers to be on hand during a disaster to help staff members work through their emotions and provide counseling.

Incident stress debriefing, in a variety of formats, is commonly offered to health care workers following an unusually stressful or traumatic incident. It helps them to process the associated emotions so that they can appropriately return to duty. Health care organizations should offer debriefing services to employees and should encourage or require employees to attend. This is vital not only for health care providers involved in disaster response, but also for those who stand ready to assist. Many organizations have some form of incident stress debriefing already in place and will only have to pull the reference into the EOP. Sidebar 7-5 (above) offers ideas for how leaders in a health care organization can help staff facing a stressful emergency situation.

Impact on the Organization

In addition to the stress on staff, the impact of emergencies on the operations of health care organizations is immense. The disruption to the organization's normal systems and processes is spread throughout the organization, from accounting operations to pharmacy services. Supplies must be provided as vendors struggle to meet a new level of demand. Information systems must function in what is often a less-than-optimal environment. The organizations' finances are strained as revenue declines and expenses mount. If the organization is itself the victim of a disaster and has to evacuate patients and shut down for a time, such as during a power failure resulting from hurricane-force winds or floods or a contagious bioterrorist-related death, financial losses accrue rapidly. The direct costs of treating patients immediately following an emergency and lost revenue resulting from the drop-off in business while the organization is attending to the disaster also can be significant.

For example, preliminary estimates from the Greater New York Hospital Association, issued less than a month after the September 11, 2001, attacks on the World Trade Center, indicate a loss of $340 million by New York City hospitals.[5] The losses were due to the combination of incremental emergency expenses, unreimbursed standby costs, and continuing fiscal impacts. The estimate did not include the significant cost increases that were required to meet new security and emergency management requirements. Following the hurricanes of 2004, the Florida Hospital Association reported that hospitals had more than $200 million in unexpected costs related to storm damage, lost revenues, staff overtime, and facility modifications to reduce potential damage during future storms.[6]

Common Reactions to Disasters

Though reactions to disasters can vary from one individual to another, there are common responses that are normal reactions to the abnormal events. Sometimes these stress reactions appear immediately following the disaster; in some cases, they are delayed for a few hours, a few days, weeks, or even months. Although the reactions detailed below might be normal, persons providing disaster behavioral health care services should refer an individual for services of a behavioral health care professional. These stress reactions can be categorized as physiological, cognitive/intellectual, emotional, and behavioral symptoms and can include the following[7,8]:

Physiological Symptoms: fatigue, nausea, headaches, vomiting, chills, ticks, teeth grinding, muscle aches, dizziness, profuse sweating, fine motor tremors

Cognitive/Intellectual Symptoms: memory loss, concentration problems, distractibility, reduced attention span, decision-making and problem-solving difficulties, calculation difficulties, and difficulty communicating thoughts, remembering instructions

Emotional Symptoms: anxiety, feeling overwhelmed, grief, identification with victims, depression, anticipation of harm to self or others, irritability, frustration

Behavioral Symptoms: disorientation, confusion, insomnia, being uncharacteristically argumentative, unnecessarily taking risks, crying easily, substance abuse, gallows humor, gait change, ritualistic behavior, hypervigilance, unwillingness to leave the scene

Coordinating with the Media

Patients will not be the only ones arriving at health care organizations in the wake of an emergency. The media also will frequently be on site, seeking information. Add to the mix volunteers wanting to help and concerned family members. Staff should be educated on strategies to handle an influx of people during an emergency. For example, staff should be trained to refer the media to the individual designated to provide them with information and direct them to an area away from patient or resident care areas as well as areas where concerned family members might be gathered.

Case Example: Florida's Quadruple Strike of Hurricanes Generates Solid Response Strategies

During a six-week period in August through September 2004, four major hurricanes tracked through coastal and central Florida, resulting in significant loss of life and numerous injuries and causing an unprecedented amount of damage to the area's critical infrastructure, property, and environment. Every health care organization in the region was, in a sense, a storm center, coping with a sudden influx of disaster victims, facility damage, staff shortages, and a myriad of other consequences.

For lessons learned from these devastating hurricanes, staff in two organizations that sustained heavy damages and faced enormous challenges were interviewed: (1) DeSoto Memorial Hospital (DeSoto), a facility with 49 beds located in rural Arcadia, and (2) Health First, an integrated delivery system with three acute care hospitals—Holmes Regional Medical Center, a 514-bed Level II trauma facility in Melbourne; the 150-bed Cape Canaveral Hospital; and the 60-bed Palm Bay Community Hospital.

Elizabeth Jordan, R.N., Ph.D., vice president of patient care services and chief nursing officer of DeSoto; Robin Bledsoe, R.N., nursing supervisor of DeSoto; and James C. Kendig, vice president of safety, security, parking, and clinical transportation of Health First, offered the following seven strategies for preparing for and responding to hurricanes and other types of emergencies.

Learn the Language and Players

At night of the day Hurricane Charley hit, DeSoto received a call through the area's emergency management system, inquiring whether the hospital needed a disaster medical assistance team (DMAT). "We thought we had to specify the types of personnel we needed, rather than just responding, 'Yes,' resulting in the delayed dispatch of needed DMAT personnel and supplies," says Jordan. In another incident, a team from Disaster Aid Services to Hospitals was turned away at the county border because officials were not familiar with that agency. "We were talking with dozens of federal, state, and local agencies, all of whom have their own language, some of which we didn't understand. I would advise colleagues to ask probing questions if they don't understand an agency's emergency response language." Participation in communitywide emergency management planning of key preparedness and response partners, including local government, fire safety, law enforcement, emergency medical services, public health, utilities, and health facilities would prevent such problems.

Participate in Communitywide Planning

Following Charley, Brevard County's Emergency Operations Center (EOC) provided a seat for a hospital representative at the ESF#8 table (Emergency Support Functions: public health and medical services). The representative met twice daily with hospital CEOs in the region to obtain information on bed, building, and operations status by organization, to learn of any issues that needed to be resolved, and to communicate communitywide information of importance to the hospitals. "This worked phenomenally well because the hospital rep could resolve hospital issues at the EOC by simply walking over to the appropriate ESF desk (for example, law enforcement, public works, transportation) to request needed resources or other help, and then report back to the hospitals at the next briefing session," says Kendig, whose organization provided the representative during Hurricane Frances. Bledsoe advises smaller organizations as follows: "Know your community's emergency management system and its planned response. Make sure you have a representative at the community's emergency management planning table, are involved in drills, and communicate frequently with potential response partners."

(continued)

Case Example: Florida's Quadruple Strike of Hurricanes Generates Solid Response Strategies, *continued*

Prepare Staff

Staff absences following hurricanes several years earlier had taught First Health the importance of conducting annual education programs to prepare all staff members for their roles and responsibilities during hurricanes. Based on a study's conclusion that stated, "It is not sufficient for a few key officials and planners to know their roles and responsibilities during a disaster, but that the roles of everyone involved must be clearly understood,"[1] Health First developed a hurricane preparedness program. It starts in January of each year, with meetings attended by representatives from all organization levels and chaired by Kendig. May is "Hurricane Preparedness Month," when each staff member receives education and a handbook covering information on staff responsibilities in pre-storm, storm, and post-storm periods; storm communication; safety; sheltering; preparation of work areas; what to bring when reporting to work; policies regarding pets; assistance available after the storm; and other topics.

Anticipate Power and Water Problems

Emergency preparedness planning identifies problems that might occur during disasters and develops strategies to prevent such problems or mitigate their impact. Loss of electrical power and water supply are common occurrences during hurricanes. "Because Charley took a different-than-expected path, Desoto had less than 45 minutes of warning for the storm. However, during this period, one of our maintenance supervisors had the foresight to turn on our emergency generator and activate our well," says Jordan. The community lost its water and power supply for weeks, but the hospital was able to provide basic life-sustaining services. "Most hospitals don't have their own wells, but they need to consider what they will do if they can't rely on tankers of water being brought to them, the backup cited in so many emergency plans. Backup to backup plans was critical for us because we were totally cut off from all supplies," comments Jordan.

Coping with the loss of nonpotable water was more of a problem in many of the affected hospitals than the loss of potable water, which was more easily brought in from the outside. To meet critical nonpotable water needs, including equipment cooling and sanitary/sewer operations, organizations might wish to consider developing a "plug-and-play" type of capability that would connect nonpotable water lines to alternative water supply from tanker trucks, existing wells, or other sources.

Both Jordan and Kendig urge organizations to "beef up" as much emergency electrical power as possible, thereby providing redundancy that could be critical. Emergency generator capabilities at DeSoto exceed those defined by *Life Safety Code®** requirements, and Health First is adding more generators at its smaller hospitals. Based on the number of stories in a building and the amount of traffic any one elevator can reasonably handle, hospitals should consider the adequacy of elevators running on generator power. To effectively continue operations with one or a limited number of functioning elevators, hospitals must address how to control elevator traffic through such strategies as limiting visitors and "staffing" the elevators.

Lack of emergency power to ventilation systems and rain that entered through louvers caused temperature and humidity levels to soar at numerous Florida hospitals, including Health First facilities, resulting in damaged sterile supplies and mold and mildew problems that extended recovery efforts. Portable emergency generators that can be brought in quickly by trailer or truck and connected to normal power branches should be considered.

(continued)

* *Life Safety Code* is a registered trademark of the National Fire Protection Association, Quincy, MA.

Case Example: Florida's Quadruple Strike of Hurricanes Generates Solid Response Strategies, *continued*

Address Care Challenges

Small, isolated DeSoto faced the challenge of providing care to 35 then-current patients and more than 300 victims who arrived within three hours in a mostly roofless and totally windowless facility. "Evacuation was not an option because there was nowhere to go," says Jordan. Staff moved inpatients down numerous flights of stairs to the center of the building's first floor, tucking each patient's medical record under his or her arm. "Our mantra was, 'Babies with their mothers, and charts with their patients,'" says Jordan. Bledsoe had already developed a plan to provide medical management from a remote site, so she put the plan into action. Runners brought medication orders to the third-floor pharmacy supply area, where the pharmacist supplied medications, and returned them back downstairs to be administered to patients. In the first hours of the storm, all internal and communication systems were severely affected, and external communication systems were knocked out, so the hospital used runners widely to communicate critical information. Bledsoe encourages health care organizations to consider numerous methods for meeting internal communication needs in the event of total communication system failure.

Approximately 10 patients who arrived at DeSoto during the hurricane in critical condition were stabilized and flown out the first evening by helicopter—the only way to access the hospital. Staffing shortages were acute for many months. Health First hospitals, which had greater available resources during the hurricanes, reduced census as low as possible prior to the storms and supported their special needs shelters for area residents who had nonurgent medical care needs. Kendig urges organizations to develop plans for the evacuation of not only patients but also ancillary support supplies. "Consider issues such as surgical supplies, blood products, and pharmaceuticals that could be damaged or rendered useless by moisture or the lack of refrigeration," says Kendig.

Meet Staff and Security Needs

Shortages are particularly challenging for staff during emergencies. "If relief staff cannot reach the facility, organizations need to consider how to meet staff respite needs. Our staff had to sleep on floors in two- to three-hour shifts for many nights," says Jordan. "Physician staff checked in and out of respite areas with a member of the medical staff office so we were aware at all times of the number and type of specialists available in our hospitals," says Kendig. Respite areas can be preplanned, but alternatives must be available in case the emergency damages intended locations.

Staff and family support needs must be addressed. "Charley severely stretched all coping skills of Arcadia residents; the sequence of three hurricanes following Charley was catastrophic. Approximately 80% of hospital employees either lost homes or had severely damaged homes; 1 in 10 staff members left the area," says Jordan. Bledsoe encourages organizations to provide staff with critical incident stress management training or to partner in the provision of such training with another hospital. "Post-traumatic stress disorder was widespread in Florida. Mental health services, in short supply nationwide, was one of the last resources we received, she says. Health First and DeSoto provided staff with such services as day care, cash advances, food and shelter, tarps for the roofs of and assistance in repairing their damaged homes, and counseling. These efforts helped to retain staff during and following the emergency.

Staff, family, and patient security issues also must be addressed. Health First controlled facility access by setting up check-in stations; requiring staff, volunteers, and families entering the building to wear predistributed wristbands; and regularly updating the inventory of building occupants.

(continued)

Case Example: Florida's Quadruple Strike of Hurricanes Generates Solid Response Strategies, *continued*

Practice, Practice, and Learn

"Drills are very good things," says Bledsoe. "So is drawing on staff's collective disaster planning and response experience while in the midst of an emergency," comments Jordan. "No one particular preparation activity met all the needs we faced, but pieces of each of them became part of the knowledge base from which we drew," says Jordan. She encourages organizations to do all they can to make drills and preparation activities "second nature." "The hurricanes presented a disaster of unbelievable magnitude for DeSoto. The staff of this small, rural hospital rose to a level of heroism that is almost impossible to describe, and the staff is still dealing with the emergency's aftermath without missing a beat," she concludes.

Reference

1. French E.D., Sole L.M., Byers J.F.: A comparison of nurses' needs/concerns and hospital disaster plans following Florida's Hurricane Floyd. *J Emerg Nurs* 28:111–117, Apr. 2002.

Source: Adapted from Joint Commission Resources: Lessons learned from Hurricanes Charley, Frances, Ivan, and Jeanne. *Environment of Care News* 8:10, Oct. 2005.

References

1. National Center for PTSD: *Disaster Rescue and Response Workers.* http://www.ncptsd.org (accessed Nov. 19, 2007).
2. Stein B.D., et al.: Emotional and behavioral consequences of bioterrorism: Planning a public health response. *Milbank Q* 82(3):413–455, 2004.
3. Landesman L.Y.: *Public Health Management of Disasters: The Practice Guide.* Washington, DC: American Public Health Association, 2001.
4. U.S. Department of Health and Human Services, Substance Abuse and Mental Health Services Administration: *Tips for Managing and Preventing Stress: A Guide for Emergency and Disaster Response Workers.* http://www.mentalhealth.samhsa.gov/publications/allpubs/KEN-01-0098/ (accessed Nov. 19, 2007).
5. Greater New York Hospital Association: *GNYHA Estimates $340 Million Loss to Hospitals Stemming from World Trade Center Attacks.* Oct. 15, 2001. http://gnyha.org/2361/Default.aspx (accessed Mar. 10, 2008).
6. Florida Hospital Association: *Eye of the Storm: Impact of the 2004 Hurricane Season on Florida Hospitals.* May 2005. http://www.fha.org/hurricanesurveyexec.pdf (accessed Feb. 12, 2008).
7. New York Office of Mental Health: *Crisis Counseling Guide to Children and Families in Disasters.* http://www.eird.org/herramientas/eng/documents/emergency/education/crisisguide.pdf (accessed Mar. 25, 2008).
8. The Center for Mental Health Services, Department of Health and Human Services: *Self-Care Tips for Emergency and Disaster Response Workers.* http://mentalhealth.samhsa.gov/publications/allpubs/KEN-01-0098/default.asp (accessed Mar. 10, 2008).

Additional Resources

Some organizations might decide to send staff to seminars offered by various health care associations. For example, the American College of Emergency Physicians has a training program for mass-casualty preparedness. The Society of Critical Care Medicine offers a course titled "Hospital Mass-Casualty Disaster Management" that addresses basic and essential disaster medical knowledge for critical care professionals. The federal Agency for Healthcare Research and Quality offers a course on emergency and disaster preparedness, as well as a free series of five Web-assisted audioconferences on bioterrorism and health system preparedness. For nurses, the American Red Cross and Sigma Theta Tau International sponsor a free two-hour online program, "Disaster Preparedness and Response for Nurses." The American Medical Association and the National Disaster Life Support Foundation also have jointly fielded a family of courses that offer instruction related to minimal to advanced disaster knowledge.

Information related to decontamination training is also available from a number of sources, such as the following:

- OSHA offers a complete list of best practices for hospital-based first receivers through its Web site, http://www.osha.gov/dts/osta/bestpractices/html/hospital_firstreceivers.html.
- The Agency for Toxic Substances and Disease Registry's Medical Management Guidelines for Acute Chemical Exposure are available on the agency's Web site at http://www.atsdr.cdc.gov/mmg.html#bookmark03.
- Organizations developing a decontamination curriculum can also look to the HazMat for Healthcare Web site (http://www.hazmatforhealthcare.org), which offers four four-hour training modules intended to help hospitals improve hazardous materials emergency response programs both for internal spills and for managing contaminated patients.
- The Environmental Protection Agency provides a four-hour decontamination program that can be offered without cost. For more information, visit the agency's Web site at http://www.epa.gov.

For information about the Centers for Disease Control and Prevention's (CDC) recommendations on how to clean and disinfect environmental surfaces, environmental sampling, laundry and bedding, and regulated medical waste, visit its Web site at http://www.cdc.gov. In addition, the Society for Healthcare Epidemiology of America, in conjunction with the CDC, offers many courses in health care epidemiology; *see* http://apic.org.

Professional organizations and state and federal agencies can provide information on organizations and individuals equipped to help staff cope with the emotional effects of trauma following a disaster.

The following organizations provide information on the psychological consequences of disasters. This list is in no way comprehensive, but is intended as a starting point for obtaining information on this subject.

- American Academy of Child and Adolescent Psychiatry: http://www.aacap.org/
- American Academy of Experts in Traumatic Stress: http://www.aaets.org/
- American Psychiatric Association: http://www.psych.org
- American Psychological Association: http://apa.org
- American Red Cross: http:/www.redcross.org
- The Center for Mental Health Services: http://mentalhealth.samhsa.gov/cmhs/
- Depression and Bipolar Support Alliance: http://www.dbsalliance.org
- Disaster Mental Health Institute at the University of South Dakota: http://www.usd.edu/dmhi/
- Disaster Technical Assistance Center: http://mentalhealth.samhsa.gov/dtac/
- Federal Emergency Management Agency: http://www.fema.gov/
- International Critical Incident Stress Foundation, Inc.: http://www.icisf.org/
- National Alliance for the Mentally Ill: http://www.nami.org/
- National Association of Social Workers: http://www.socialworkers.org/
- National Center for Posttraumatic Stress Disorder: http://www.ncptsd.va.gov/ncmain/index.jsp
- National Institute of Mental Health: http://www.nimh.nih.gov/
- National Mental Health Association: http://www.nmha.org/

Chapter 8

Establishing Strategies for Managing Utilities

Utilities are essential to the proper operation of the environment of care and significantly contribute to effective, safe, and reliable care. Yet utilities are often one of the first losses during internal or external emergencies, both natural and man-made. Managing essential utilities—the functioning of an organization's electricity, water, fuel, ventilation, and so forth—in the face of an emergency must not be compromised or adverse events could occur. This chapter, as detailed in Sidebar 8-1, addresses the importance of planning for alternative means for providing the following:

- Electrical power
- Water
- Fuel
- Other needs—ventilation, medical gas, vacuum systems

Managing Utilities

Different types of emergencies can have the same detrimental impact on an organization's utility systems. For example, hurricanes and earthquakes could both knock out electricity. Or, flooding could interrupt water service. In 2003 something as innocuous as a falling tree limb cut power lines in Ohio and knocked out power across a swath of New England and the Mid-Atlantic states.[1]

No matter the emergency, the loss of utilities in itself can create an emergency for health care organizations. The need to plan for utility requirements during an emergency has long been part of Joint Commission emergency management standards and environment of care standards and is now given special emphasis as one of the six critical functions.

The loss of utilities is not uncommon during emergencies. Disasters such as ice storms, hurricanes, and tornadoes can all result in loss of utilities required for care, treatment, and services. Organizations should identify alternative means of providing for essential utilities. The standard under discussion breaks down these utilities into greater detail by separating water into potable (for consumption and care) and non-potable sources (for equipment and sanitation).

Sidebar 8-1.
Applicable Emergency Management Standard

The organization establishes strategies for managing utilities during emergencies.

This standard requires the following:
Organizations identify an alternative means of providing for the following utilities in the event that their supply is compromised or disrupted:

1. Electricity
2. Water needed for consumption and essential care activities
3. Water needed for equipment and sanitary purposes
4. Fuel required for building operations or essential transport activities
5. Other essential utility needs (for example, ventilation, medical gas/vacuum systems)

Key questions to consider for utility failure might include the following:

- Does your organization's emergency management plan address how the organization would handle a utility failure caused by an interruption in service by a utility provider? A lightning strike?
- What effect would a utility failure have on your organization? How has your emergency management plan addressed such effects?
- What backup systems are in place in the event of a utility failure?

Facilities must identify alternative means of meeting essential building utility needs when the facility must provide continuous service during an emergency. Electricity, water, ventilation, fuel sources, and medical gas/vacuum systems might each require special consideration. For example, organizations must consider supplemental emergency generators, the operation of emergency generators, the placement of emergency generators to protect them from potential hazards as well as theft, and other critical equipment. Generators and the fuel necessary to power them should be situated so that they are not at risk from flooding. In addition to placing generators above possible flood zones, it is important to ensure that switching components necessary to go from normal electrical operations to generator operations are not located in low-lying areas.[2] Organizations should also consider what happens if the generator designed to serve as a backup also fails. Most generators are not designed to power a facility for extended periods of time.[2] Having parts to repair a broken-down generator could make a difference in the success or failure of the emergency operations plan (EOP). In essence, utility management issues come down to contingency planning.

Be Prepared Tip

Information Technology Needs

If information technology is part of emergency operations considerations, is it included on the electrical backup systems? Are the computers that need to access the system also on the backup systems?[1]

Reference

1. American Health Lawyers Association: *Emergency Preparedness, Response & Recovery Checklist: Beyond the Emergency Management Plan.* Washington, DC: American Health Lawyers Association, 2004.

To address the need for water, many organizations plan for tankers of water to be brought to the facility if normal sources are not available. Organizations should consider, though, what will happen if the tankers cannot arrive due to blocked roads. To meet the need for water required for equipment and sanitary and sewer operations, one approach is to develop a "plug-and-play" capability that connects nonpotable water lines to alternative water supplies from tanker trucks, existing wells, or other sources.[3]

One organization that was hit by Hurricane Katrina also found that its plans for nonpotable water necessary to wash floors did not work as planned. Trash cans used to collect water came apart under the weight of the water, and the organization was forced to clean its floors with alcohol and peroxide.[4] This shows the need to consider how nonpotable water for cleaning, equipment, and toilets will be collected and stored.

To prepare for a utility failure, an organization's EOP should outline procedures for the following:

- Prompt repair or replacement
- Provision of appropriate alternative clinical care so that little or no increase in risk to care recipients occurs during failure
- The partial or total cessation of services
- The possible evacuation of care recipients in the event of a prolonged system outage

Organizations should identify alternative means of providing for essential utilities, whether through negotiated relationships with primary suppliers, memoranda of understanding with other organizations, redundant or alternative equipment at the organization, or provision through a parent entity. Organizations should also consider how they would address utilities management if community resources were not available. They should not rely solely on single-source providers in the community but should identify other suppliers outside the local community.

To ensure that utilities will be available during an emergency, an organization must have accurate and current contingency plans. These plans should be exercised or confirmed to ensure that the system will be reliable. Without these tests, the risk of failure is unknown.

Be Prepared Tip

Know the Facility

Organizations should understand clearly which parts of the facility are served by generators, as well as how the water system works. If the water supply is disrupted or polluted, water use might need to be limited in order to conserve scarce supplies. And water pumped from wells might not be available without electricity.

Coordinating with the Media

Organizations should be prepared to communicate with the media about utilities. During the early stages of an emergency, the media might wish to know if utilities are still functioning. This provides an opportunity to explain that the organization has plans for alternatives that will ensure that essential utilities are available to care for patients. If utility failures occur, the organization should provide the most up-to-date information about the situation and how it is being handled.

In health care organizations that establish their own media center, organizations should consider what types of utilities will be needed. For example, electricity and wireless capabilities are basic to ensuring access to telephones, computers, faxes, modems, and so forth and might be an issue to consider in managing utilities during an emergency.

Case Example:
Lessons from One Storm and Multiple Disasters

The escalating disaster scenario of Hurricane Katrina put emergency management plans to a severe test at hospitals in New Orleans and elsewhere along the Gulf Coast in August and September 2005. One organization that was affected was Tulane University Hospital & Clinic, a 235-bed academic medical center near the Louisiana Superdome. In the chaos that was brought about by Hurricane Katrina and the subsequent flood, the hospital protected itself from widespread civil unrest, and the entire facility was successfully evacuated.

George Jamison, Tulane's director of facilities management and a *Life Safety Code*®* Specialist, played a key role in the hospital's emergency response. Shortly after the evacuation, Jamison described 10 lessons learned from the multiple disasters brought about by the storm. The 10 lessons cover aspects across all of the Joint Commission's emergency management standards, including managing utilities as described in Lesson 7. Although Hurricane Katrina left behind incredible damage, it also yielded important information about how health care organizations can make sure they are ready for escalating and multiple disasters.

1. Invest in the planning process.

Jamison says conducting hazard vulnerability analyses (HVAs) and developing a written emergency management plan have been among the hospital's top priorities. "We update our HVA every six months when we do our Statement of Conditions™," he says. Because of the risks identified in an HVA, the hospital augmented its stock of emergency items

(continued)

* *Life Safety Code* is a registered trademark of the National Fire Protection Association, Quincy, MA.

Case Example: Lessons from One Storm and Multiple Disasters, *continued*

such as pumps, sandbags, and inflatable door dams—items that proved essential in the disaster. Jamison says effort put into the emergency management plan paid off as well: "Staff were familiar with it and they did it. This experience shows that the more you put into the planning process, the more you get out of it.

"One thing hospitals need to tighten up on is actually 'walking out' their plan." Jamison encourages facilities managers to test their plans physically: "Walk to the triage area, walk to the decontamination area," he says. "You may even want to make a video of it to show during orientation." Jamison also recommends exercising contingency plans, particularly regarding utility systems. He places particular importance on shutoff valves; you should not only identify your main valves but operate them as part of regular testing.

2. Realize you might have to go it alone.

As part of its disaster planning program, Tulane established links with both the community at large and neighboring health care organizations. However, because the Katrina disaster was so widespread, these resources did not ultimately prove useful. In addition, police and public utility support were limited or nonexistent through much of the crisis. Although government and peer backup is a legitimate element of any emergency plan, Katrina showed the importance of mapping out an extra layer of protection for handling extreme and escalating situations.

"It's not so much the situation," says Jamison, "it's how you handle it." He notes that stocking up on emergency supplies is important; Tulane had food and water for five days and pharmaceutical supplies for seven days. Jamison also advocated establishing dependable relationships with key suppliers.

3. Exercise to the breaking point.

If Hurricane Katrina proved anything, it is that disasters do not always come in neat, single packages. New Orleans experienced not one disaster scenario but four—hurricane, flooding, utilities failure, and civil disturbance. "During Katrina, we had a series of multiple events," says Jamison. "I think the only way you can be prepared for that is to exercise it."

When conducting emergency management exercises, says Jamison, organizations should simulate the domino effect of actual disasters—sequential failures in power, communication, equipment, and so forth. "When you are exercising your emergency plan, your aim should be to stress the plan until it breaks. This is the real world." He says that instead of demoralizing staff, exercising to failure actually makes them more confident. "When you exercise to one thing after another, people learn they can always find a way to deal with the situation."

4. Establish command.

Jamison believes the most important lessons from Hurricane Katrina is "the three Cs"—command, control, and communicate. "Set up command, control it, and communicate it," he says. "If you do that, everything else will fit into place."

Jamison says Tulane's command model, a modified version of the Hospital Incident Command Systems, worked exceptionally well during the crisis. He cautions that organizations need to ensure that several backup people understand the emergency plan and be able to implement it. He also stresses the importance of identifying alternative roles and reporting lines within the command structure. One strength of the plan is that it clarifies the role of physicians, who are organized into teams under the chief medical officer. Jamison says assigning staff to cover essential functions took place early in the disaster response.

(continued)

Case Example: Lessons from One Storm and Multiple Disasters, *continued*

One way to support the command function is to create a condensed version of the emergency management plan that can be used for instant reference during a crisis. Tulane's condensed plan document includes key information broken out into bullet points.

5. Establish control.

Controlling the situation is always important during an emergency. In the aftermath of Katrina, it became a serious issue. Following the storm, it was critically important to limit and screen persons entering the hospital (including new patients). Jamison says emergency plans should map out all possible entrances. At Tulane, armed security staff acted quickly to lock down and guard entrance points. Internal security was also an issue; officers had to isolate and closely monitor certain individuals who threatened trouble.

Other aspects of control are maintaining fire safety (the hospital organized six two-person fire watch patrols) and handling the media. At one point, Jamison had to insist that a national television news crew follow his safety-related orders or leave the facility.

Jamison says that one of the most effective tools for maintaining control is giving key staffers badges identifying them as safety officers. "Any kind of badge of authority means a lot," he says. "When you're wearing a badge, people come up to you and ask what's happening and what you want them to do."

6. Communicate.

During the Katrina crisis, Jamison found that communication is half the battle. One element is having processes in place for communicating with patients. According to Jamison, patient communication during the crisis was "mouth to ear"—a hospital leader gave regular briefings to ambulatory patients, and then nurses carried key information to inpatients. Jamison says staff communication was also a priority. "Every five hours, we mustered the entire staff, everyone from the VP to the floor cleaners," he says. "We let them know what was happening, what they could expect, and what we wanted from them."

Katrina inflicted heavy damage on many hospitals' communication technologies—the storm not only downed telephone lines, it also ripped off the radio antennas from some of the hospitals' roofs. In addition, cell phones became inoperable. Fortunately, Tulane staff were ably to amplify the signal of a satellite telephone to achieve outside communication. It is important for organizations to reexamine the integrity of their backup communication systems. As the result of Katrina, Jamison planned to install a removable radio antenna that can be taken down before a storm and put up again after the winds have died down. The organization also found that it needed to train staff members in the use of basic radio equipment.

7. Take a hard look at utilities.

Joint Commission standards require health care organizations to plan alternative means of meeting essential building utility needs. Tulane's experience shows that ensuring utility backup requires foresight and creativity.

Jamison says Tulane's main emergency generator was vulnerable to flooding during the disaster. What saved the hospital were its portable generator sets, which could be moved to safe positions. Portable generators were able to support ventilators for critically ill patients. In addition, engineering staff had previously constructed portable power panels that provided flexibility in addressing electricity needs. Staff met fuel needs by siphoning gasoline from cars left in the hospital's parking structure.

(continued)

Case Example: Lessons from One Storm and Multiple Disasters, *continued*

Although expensive, positioning main generator units higher could be considered a priority for health care organizations in flood zones. Jamison says that when Katrina hit, Tulane had just committed the funds for putting two generators on the second floor of the parking structure.

Jamison notes that one utility issue often overlooked is sewer service. Prior to Katrina, he had obtained 1,500 pounds of cat litter. To help control rising sewage, bags of the material were placed around toilets in the days before the storm. Later, after sewer service was knocked out, the litter was used in the toilets. "It absorbs 80% of its weight," says Jamison. "You put two cups of it in a red bag and place it in the bowl." This method helped ensure sanitation throughout the crisis.

8. Plan seriously for an evacuation.

For most health care organizations, the primary strategy for responding to an emergency is "defend in place." Hurricane Katrina showed that this cannot be the only strategy, as do the emergency management standards. At Tulane, utilities failures, limited supplies, and civil unrest forced the command team to order an evacuation a day after serious flooding began.

Jamison and his crew created a helicopter landing pad on the top level of the parking structure by taking down light poles and painting large yellow arrows. The organization had determined that the structure would support a helicopter's weight. In accordance with the emergency management standard, the emergency plan included processes for tracking evacuated patients. When a helicopter arrived, a coordinator at the pad called down to the triage center for a specified number of patients. Nursing staff matched charts to wristbands and sent the requested patients up, sometimes with medications and intravenous apparatus. As a final check, an associate vice president stationed on the roof did a final confirmation before the patient was loaded onto the helicopter and flown to the preplanned alternative care site.

9. Plan to lock down.

In an evacuation, the main priority is getting everyone out safely. A complete emergency response, however, also includes strategies for mitigation and recovery. Jamison says it is crucial to secure potentially dangerous materials and take steps to support recovery. "If you can leave on your own terms, you will be better off," he says. "Our approach was to secure anything that people could use to hurt themselves, hurt others, or sell on the black market."

Jamison also took several steps to support the eventual recovery efforts. Staff stayed on top of garbage control—compartmentalizing trash in designated sections of the hospital during the crisis and continuing to bag garbage even as the evacuation drew to a close. Staffers also opened certain windows for ventilation. Before evacuating, Jamison and his crew disconnected breakers and demagnetized and degaussed MRI equipment. The bottom line: Minimize damage to the facility and enable a future reoccupation.

10. Rethink plans for family of staff.

In keeping with another Joint Commission standard, emergency management plans commonly include provisions for supporting family members of essential staff. Under normal circumstances, Tulane's approach—arranging discounted rates for family members at a nearby hotel—is a reasonable arrangement. The civil unrest following Hurricane Katrina, however, put everyone in serious danger.

(continued)

Case Example: Lessons from One Storm and Multiple Disasters, *continued*

Jamison says that although concern about family did not keep his staff from doing their jobs, it did slow them down. "It was hard, but this is probably the most awesome staff I have ever had." He said the experience was a sobering lesson for everyone. In light of it, health care organizations saw a need to rethink their strategies for ensuring the safety of family members during an emergency.

Not if, but when

Jamison says the biggest challenges of Katrina came not from the hurricane itself but from the aftermath. "We have 12 or 15 storms a year," says Jamison. "It's not a matter of if a storm will hit but when it will hit and how severe it will be."

No matter their location, all health care organizations can benefit by taking a similar attitude toward emergency management. Katrina showed that organizations need to make the worst-case scenario part of their emergency plans. The only way to survive an emergency is to expect it.

Source: Reprinted from Joint Commission Resources: 10 lessons from escalating disasters. *Environment of Care News* 9:2, Feb. 2006.

Case Example: Contingency Plans for Utility Systems

It's a Sunday evening in January, and your organization is weathering the biggest snowstorm it has seen in years. It is 25°F (–3.9°C) outside, and the windchill factor makes it feel like –10°F (–23°C). You just got off the phone with the manager of the city's steam power plant. There has been a failure due to the weather, and the plant is temporarily off-line. Consequently, your organization is without its city-generated steam heat. Fortunately, you have a contingency plan for just this type of situation; are you confident that the contingency plan will be effective?

The answer to that question might depend on whether your organization has recently tested its steam contingency plan. For example, what if your organization's steam contingency plan involves shutting off a valve in the street behind the main facility so that steam can be diverted back into the building, and what if the valve is the same one that was installed when the building was built in 1940, and the contingency plan was created by the individual who managed utilities at the time? In other words, what if the valve has never been tested? If the valve has not been tested recently, there is a good chance that the valve will break off in your hand when you try to shut it off. Not only would this not address the lack-of-steam problem your organization is facing, it would also possibly necessitate evacuating the building to another location where there was heat. What started as a utility outage would quickly transform into a crisis for your organization.

On the other hand, if you tested the valve last summer and it worked, the probability that it will work during the crisis increases. Even if the valve didn't work during the test, but you fixed the valve before colder weather arrived, your organization would have avoided a crisis and ensured the continuation of steam heat during the snowstorm.

(continued)

Case Example: Contingency Plans for Utility Systems, *continued*

"Many organizations created contingency plans for their utilities when their buildings were new but have not exercised them since," says George Mills, F.A.S.H.E., C.E.M., C.H.E.M., senior engineer, Standards Interpretation Group, The Joint Commission. "By periodically testing utility contingency plans during controlled situations that do not negatively affect patients, staff, and visitors, organizations can avoid a crisis and ensure the continuous delivery of quality of care.

Another Joint Commission Requirement

Utility systems are essential to the proper operation of the environment of care and significantly contribute to the effective, safe, and reliable provision of care to patients in health care organizations. Although there is an emergency management standard that deals with establishing strategies for managing utilities during an emergency, there is another Joint Commission standard that also addresses an organization's readiness.

According to one environment of care standard, organizations must manage their utility risks. This management process should not only ensure the operational reliability of utility systems, but also minimize the potential risks of utility system failures. Creating and exercising contingency plans, which involve backup systems that can be used in an emergency, can help minimize potential risks during a utility failure.

According to The Joint Commission, utility systems can include any of the following:

- Electrical distribution
- Emergency power
- Vertical transport (elevators)
- Horizontal transport (pneumatic tube systems and others)
- Heating, ventilation, and air-conditioning
- Plumbing
- Boiler and steam
- Piped gases
- Vacuum systems
- Communication systems (including data exchange)

Not every health care organization will have all these systems, but for any system present, an organization should have a contingency plan in place in case the system fails.

Determining Priorities

Depending on the type of organization, there might be different utility systems present. Addressing risks and potential failures in all utility backup systems at once is not realistic due to the potential lack of resources, such as time, money, and staff. Before testing contingency plans, an organization needs to make sure it is testing the most critical plans first. For example, addressing the lack of backup steam might be more critical than addressing an issue in the backup pneumatic tube system.

"Organizations should consider conducting a proactive risk assessment, such as failure mode and effects analysis, to prioritize what needs to be addressed first," says Mills. This type of assessment can help the organization determine potential utility backup system failures, identify the risks associated with those failures, prioritize issues to be fixed, determine ways to fix the priorities, and implement solutions to avoid potentially harmful situations. "By conducting a risk analysis first,

(continued)

Case Example: Contingency Plans for Utility Systems, *continued*

organizations can address the most critical issues immediately and create a timetable for addressing other issues in the future," says Mills. (Note: The hazard vulnerability analysis process that each organization uses as part of emergency management is also relevant to this approach.)

Timing Is Everything

When testing contingency plans, timing is everything. Organizations should plan to conduct a test when the effects of a potential failure would be minimal and when the safety of patients, staff, and visitors will not be compromised. "While it is important to periodically test contingency plans, it should be done in an appropriate way that does not negatively impact safety," says Mills. "Without careful forethought and planning, an organization's test can cause more harm than good." In the case of the previously mentioned steam example, an organization could consider conducting the valve test in July, when steam heat is not needed. That way, if the valve fails, patients, staff, and visitors are not negatively affected by the failure in the backup system.

"Organizations may also want to consider testing a utility's contingency plan during an emergency management exercise. For example, if an organization is conducting an exercise that involves a loss of potable water, the organization may want to exercise the water valves at this time to see if they function and if an effective contingency plan is in place," says Mills.

Planning for Failure

Before embarking on a test of a utility's contingency plan, organizations should set aside resources to address whatever failures might be discovered during the test. For example, if your organization is going to test the previously mentioned valve to divert steam heat, you should have funds in place to replace that valve if it breaks during the test. If an organization cannot allocate sufficient funds, then plans must be made for a secondary backup to the system being tested to ensure that a loss in backup utility will not affect the environment of care (EC) or patient safety. For example, if an organization tests its emergency power system, it would be appropriate to conduct a test when an alternative generator is present or easily accessible so that any loss of emergency backup power would be for a short duration.

Involving Others in Planning

When planning a test of a utility system's contingency plan, EC professionals should discuss the test with the organization's multidisciplinary group that addresses EC issues (this group might be called the EC committee or the safety committee). "It's important that any discipline that could be affected by the test be aware of it. Also, a multidisciplinary group may help anticipate problems the EC professional might not consider," says Mills. For example, if your organization is planning to test its medical gas utility backup system, everyone in the organization who would use medical gas should be aware that the test is going on and that there is a chance that the backup system could be compromised. Organizations should schedule tests well in advance and process any requests for tests in writing, to ensure that the verification and approval of the tests are documented. Before conducting a test, an organization should make sure any backup equipment or personnel are on site and ready to step in if the backup system fails.

During an actual utility failure is not the time to discover that your contingency plan is not effective. Organizations that regularly test their contingency plans and address any problems that arise are better prepared for emergencies and increase the likelihood of preserving patient safety and quality of care.

Source: Reprinted from Joint Commission Resources: Contingency plans for utility systems. *Environment of Care News* 10:1, Jan. 2007.

For Additional Assistance

The Joint Commission offers strategies on preventing adverse events related to electrical power failures in its *Sentinel Event Alert* Issue #37, found at http://www.jointcommission.org/SentinelEvents/SentinelEventAlert/sea_37.htm.

The *Alert* was published in response to clinical operations that were negatively affected when normal power was lost during the Houston floods of 2001, the northeastern United States blackout in 2003, and major hurricanes Charlie, Francis, Ivan, and Jeanne in 2004 and Katrina and Rita in 2005.

References

1. American Health Lawyers Association: *Emergency Preparedness, Response & Recovery Checklist: Beyond the Emergency Management Plan.* Washington, DC: American Health Lawyers Association, 2004.
2. To evacuate or not to evacuate? *Healthcare Benchmarks Qual Improv* p. 125, Nov. 2005.
3. Joint Commission Resources: Lessons learned from Hurricanes Charley, Frances, Ivan, and Jeanne. *Environment of Care News* 8:10, Oct. 2005.
4. Greene J.: Katrina teaches disaster planning lessons. *OR Manager* 21:7–8, Nov. 2005.

Chapter 9

Managing Clinical and Support Activities

The clinical needs of patients during an emergency are of prime importance, and certain clinical activities are so fundamental to safe and effective care that organizations must have clear, reasonable plans in place to address the needs of patients during extreme conditions. For example, organizations should determine how they reschedule or manage clinical needs in rapidly changing situations or in an environment that hardly mirrors the normal, modern conditions of most hospitals or long term care facilities. Because emergencies are by their nature so unpredictable, organizations considering how they provide care in an emergency must think about a variety of situations that could include little or no external support or resources.

This chapter concentrates on the final critical emergency management area, the necessity of having clear and reasonable plans in place to address the needs of patients or residents when an organization's resources are taxed. Sidebar 9-1 (below) details Joint Commission expectations related to managing clinical and support activities.

Managing Clinical Activities

The fundamental goal of emergency management planning is to protect life and prevent disability. This means that organizations must consider how to provide care during dynamic situations. The standard serving as the focus of this chapter, managing clinical and support activities, includes many concepts previously found in emergency management standards, such as triage, scheduling, modifying services, and so forth, as well as a new focus on vulnerable populations, the personal hygiene and sanitation needs of patients, mental health needs, mortuary services, and documenting and tracking clinical information.

The manner in which care is provided could vary depending on the type of emergency, requiring organizations to deter-

Sidebar 9-1.

Applicable Emergency Management Standards

The organization establishes strategies for managing clinical and support activities during emergencies.

This standard requires that the organization plans to manage the following during emergencies:

- The clinical activities required as part of patient scheduling, triage, assessment, treatment, admission, transfer, discharge, and evacuation
- Clinical services for vulnerable populations served by the organization, including patients who are pediatric, geriatric, disabled, or have serious chronic conditions or addictions
- Personal hygiene and sanitation needs of its patients
- The mental health service needs of its patients
- mortuary services

The organization plans for documenting and tracking patients' clinical information.

Be Prepared Tip

Transferring

It is important that both sending and receiving physicians be involved in transferring care recipients and that all necessary documentation and records accompany the individuals. Remember that just because it is an emergency, the organization is not automatically exempt from COBRA and OBRA regulations.

mine how they will reschedule or manage clinical needs in spite of the challenges that arise during a disaster. The emergency triage process will typically result in patients being quickly treated and discharged, admitted for a longer stay, or transferred to a more appropriate source of care. It is particularly important to identify and triage patients whose clinical needs are outside the usual scope of services of the organization. A catastrophic emergency could result in a decision to keep all patients on the premises in the interest of safety, or, conversely, in the decision to evacuate all patients because the facility is no longer safe. Planning for clinical services must address these situations accordingly.

Triage and Beyond

Triage can be one of the most challenging issues associated with managing clinical and support activities. Organizations must adjust normal triage protocols when faced with an influx of individuals seeking treatment during an emergency, with a focus on rapidly identifying the critically injured. The difficulty is to identify those who are critically injured and require immediate care. An example of a triage algorithm that hospitals and long term care organizations can use during emergencies appears in Figure 9-1 at right.

By adjusting triage protocols, organizations can free up space in the facility by delaying the treatment of those who are not critically injured or ill in anticipation of more critically injured or ill victims arriving as a result of the emergency. In a hospital, the head emergency physician or surgeon might serve as a triage gatekeeper. The medical director may fulfill the same role at Medicare-/Medicaid-based long term care organizations. Involving nursing leaders also makes sense.

Organizations will probably see a large number of slightly injured patients who have not been evaluated. This first wave is generally made up of patients who are ambulatory and have

Figure 9-1. Triage Algorithm

This triage algorithm assesses the victim's ability to obey commands, the presence of respirations, and the palpability of the radial pulse.

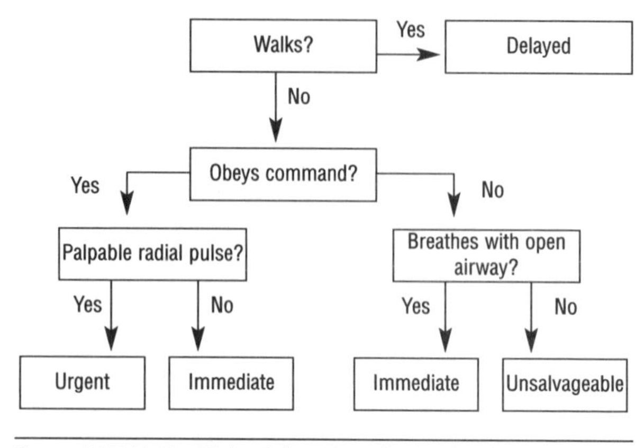

Source: NRMA CareFlight, Sydney, Australia. Used with permission.

arrived at the facility by their own means. Depending on the location of the emergency, it might be necessary to send a team to provide on-site triage. The triage area must be large enough to accommodate several response vehicles, as well as patients who arrive from the emergency scene by regular vehicles. This area should be protected from the weather as much as possible.

In an internal emergency, the emergency department (ED) is the most logical location for triage in a hospital because the personnel assigned there are experienced with rapidly evaluating and sorting a large number of patients. In the case of an external emergency, the local emergency medical services (EMS) system can provide on-site triage. Most EMS systems use color-coded tags to identify patients by severity of injury. In general, the categories are red, yellow, green, and black, as described in Table 9-1 (page 119). Red is for patients who need immediate intervention, possibly in an operating room. Yellow is for those who are seriously injured but whose care can be delayed in order to treat category-red patients. The "walking wounded" make up the green category, including patients having severe psychological reactions. The black category is reserved for the dead or those who are near death. The triage of dying patients depends on the resources available at the scene. Some systems include another category—white—used for patients with no apparent injury who are transported to a hospital for other reasons. Health care organizations should be familiar with the system used in their community.

Table 9-1. Triage Categories

The following color-coded categories are often used by emergency medical services (EMS) systems.

Red: Immediately life-threatening, could need surgical intervention. Those tagged as red are "golden-hour" trauma patients. Critical interventions have been started at the scene and need to be continued by the emergency department (ED) staff. This category could also include high-profile patients the media will be asking about.

Yellow: Serious and potentially unstable. These patients could deteriorate into category red. They have a potential threat to life or limb and will probably be admitted to the facility or be transferred to a higher-level facility when they are stable.

Green: Slightly injured. These are "walking wounded" patients—usually the majority of emergency victims—and do not have life- or limb-threatening injuries. Their injuries are of the severity commonly seen in "fast-track" areas of the ED or urgent-care centers. Keep in mind that EMS triage protocols place hysterical patients in this category, and so their needs might include pastoral care or other kinds of counseling.

Black: Dead or near death. These are the dead or dying who under ordinary circumstances would need extensive resources to stay alive. In general, out-of-hospital personnel (paramedics and emergency medical technicians) do not perform cardiopulmonary resuscitation during emergency operations.

Source: Joint Commission Resources: *Guide to Emergency Management Planning in Health Care.* Oakbrook Terrace, IL: Joint Commission on Accreditation of Healthcare Organizations, 2002.

Most hospitals then use a second round of triage at the ambulance bay of the ED. From there, medical personnel send patients to different treatment areas in the hospital: the operating room (OR), ED, ambulatory treatment area (usually a cafeteria or auditorium), or morgue. Depending on the nature of the unfolding emergency, it could be necessary to expand the treatment areas into clinics or urgent-care centers.

Studies have shown that when a moderate- to large-scale emergency happens in an urban area, the majority of victims will be treated by one or two hospitals, regardless of the number of facilities available. Often these are the hospitals known for their emergency or trauma care or even their proximity to the emergency. If a hospital under consideration is in an urban area, those in charge should plan to admit and treat patients, even if it is unlikely to be called on. First, the emergency could happen near the hospital. Second, there could be an overflow of patients diverted from other facilities. If the hospital is in a smaller community, the facility might be the only one available to receive patients, and effective preparation would be essential to save lives.

To have enough space to triage and care for emergency victims in hospitals, it might be necessary to clear out inpatient beds and the ED. The emergency operations plan (EOP) should specify how to discharge patients who are able to go home. It should also identify all the open beds in the facility, call for the immediate transfer of patients in the ED who require admission to inpatient beds with notification to their admitting physician, and outline the procedures for processing the remaining patients and the slightly injured patients who are arriving. Organizations might have to cancel elective surgeries to use OR suites and free up personnel.

In addition to scheduling and triage, along with the assessment that occurs as part of the triage process, organizations must also consider how they will handle admission and discharge. In essence, all of the processes that occur on a routine basis must be considered under emergency conditions. In addition, how will the organization manage clinical needs if an evacuation is necessary?

Emergent and urgent conditions will continue to present in the daily population the hospital or long term care organization services, and so there must be procedures to handle the ongoing flow of individuals to the facility. In addition, a severe emergency can disrupt the local care network. The organization could become the primary care provider for individuals whose primary care physicians are not available because of displacement or injury. Many types of injuries (sprain, puncture wounds, lacerations, falls) occur during emergency recovery phases as people clear debris and rebuild their homes. Due to fuels used for heating and cooking, there can be cases of carbon monoxide exposure. Health care organizations must anticipate and plan for providing an increased amount of primary care both during and following an emergency.

People with Special Needs

People with special needs include not only the vulnerable elderly but also people with disabilities, such as individuals who are physically challenged; people with sensory limitations such as the blind or visually impaired and those who are deaf or severely hard of hearing; people with severe emotional impairments; people with medically related needs, such as those who require dialysis; individuals with seizure disorders; and many others who require unique assistance.[1] The Web site of the National Rehabilitation Information Center (http://www.naric.com) provides contact information on a number of organizations composed of people with special needs.

Reference

1. Federal Emergency Management Agency: *Individuals with Special Needs: Preparing and Planning.* http://www.fema.gov/plan/prepare/specialplans.shtm (accessed Nov. 28, 2007).

Vulnerable Populations

Properly treating special needs populations during an emergency or disaster requires special planning. One of the new requirements related to the managing clinical and support activities standard is that organizations must plan to manage services for vulnerable populations served, including those who are pediatric, geriatric, disabled, or have serious chronic conditions or addictions. The need to consider special populations was made clear in the aftermath of Hurricane Katrina, which claimed as victims 34 residents of a nursing home located on the outskirts of New Orleans.[1] In addition to those who are already in the hospital or long term care facility when the emergency occurs, this new requirement related to vulnerable populations includes those in the community who might come into contact with the organization as the emergency develops.

Vulnerable populations such as the elderly, the disabled, children, and others with special needs often require special attention or assistance in emergency situations. Organizations should encourage health practitioners to attend training sessions that teach the appropriate management of life-threatening events in the special populations as well as address assessment, appropriate triaging issues, and management of populations with special needs.

Children are included in this Joint Commission requirement because the differences in pediatric patients from the adult population are many and can come into play in an emergency situation. For example, children cannot be decontaminated in decontamination units designed for adults; young people are more vulnerable than adults to chemical agents that are absorbed through the skin or that are inhaled; and young people are more susceptible than adults to dehydration, shock from biological agents, and radiation exposure.[2] EMS and ED staff should have the necessary training to treat these patients with the appropriate interventions in case of an emergency.

Be Prepared Tip

Assess the Population and Identify the Most Vulnerable

Hospitals and long term care organizations seeking to meet the vulnerable populations component of the emergency management standards should consider both physical and cognitive limitations. Cognitive impairments could limit a person's ability to follow directions, and changes in routine could result in anxiety and disruptive behaviors. A physical limitation might require use of a wheelchair, special transportation, or life-sustaining treatments, for example.

In addition, the developmental abilities and cognitive levels of children might impede their ability to escape danger. Children also have unique psychological vulnerabilities, so special management plans are needed in the event of mass casualties and evacuation.[2]

The American Academy of Pediatrics (AAP) recommends that hospitals incorporate appropriate types and numbers of pediatric-trained staff, equipment, medications, and decontamination equipment, including the ability to handle nonambulatory children, into their EOPs. In addition, the AAP says, hospitals must be prepared to handle situations in which patients will be cared for as a family unit and children will not be able to be separated from adults, such as in a quarantine situation.

Be Prepared Tip

Gathering Input on Vulnerable Populations

Meeting the needs of vulnerable populations can be more manageable by focusing on the formation of committee made up of the larger community that include elderly persons and those with special needs (and their advocates) to gain direct input concerning priorities, necessary accommodations, and appropriate services for emergency situations. In addition, organizations can help special populations understand their roles in emergency situations. For example, this could include encouraging patients through efforts such as the Joint Commission's Speak Up™ campaign to ask questions and demand answers about emergency planning. Engaging patients in the process can help organizations determine how effectively their message is being received.

This requires hospitals to have the capability to handle children and for children's hospitals to be able to care for adult patients who would stay with their children. To ensure that these pediatric needs are adequately considered, hospitals should be sure to include pediatricians and emergency pediatricians in their emergency management planning, training, and drills.[3]

In long term care settings, the emphasis on disaster management is on the population served if it is an internal disaster. However, in a community emergency, the organization must also be prepared for walk-ins. Every long term care organization must be prepared to move patients from one facility to another or, in the event of a community disaster, to locations far away. It could also mean that care is provided in austere care environments. This requires a systematic and redundant plan that takes into account individual needs, such as ensuring that patients' medication regiment is not disrupted in an emergency evacuation or that sensory aids such as eyeglasses, hearing aids, and so forth, are accounted for.

Effective emergency management also depends on strong relationships among health care organizations and the community at large. Regional partnerships must be built and maintained to integrate planned responses before an emergency or a disaster occurs. This is particularly important when the emergency involves a special population such as the vulnerable elderly. In the case of a communitywide emergency, all health care organizations might be needed—whether to assist with triage and urgent care of victims, provide nonurgent care to others, shelter community members or patients from other facilities that have been evacuated, or supply specific staff and/or supplies to other organizations.[4]

As discussed in Chapter 7, it is important that organizations include emergency preparedness in new employee orientation programs to ensure that new staff understand the various populations concerned, the identified vulnerabilities, and the system of response in a variety of cases. This applies to both front-line staff and to leadership. Emergency preparation is an ongoing process for staff and patients alike, and training staff to assist those with special needs must include instruction on such issues as transporting, lifting or carrying, and communicating with these individuals. It can also be valuable to include advocates or those with special needs themselves in the training process.[4]

Organizations should also be prepared to address the aftereffects of a traumatic event by providing resources on mental health and recovery, as well as educational materials that review how to recognize and monitor the acute and longer-term psychological impact of disaster events. Although children might need special attention after an emergency, organizations should also consider how other vulnerable populations, such as the elderly, disabled, or those with serious chronic conditions or addictions, might need similar help after an emergency.

Finally, addressing the needs of vulnerable populations can go both ways. Hospitals and long term care organizations should encourage independent and community-based individuals with special needs to carry with them information explaining their conditions and special instructions for assistance or treatment; a list of their medications, allergies, sensitivities, and requisite special equipment; and the names and telephone numbers of their physicians and family contacts. Community-based individuals with special needs should be encouraged to have a support network of family or friends who will assist them in an emergency.[4] Sidebar 9-2 (page 122) provides information on how organizations can help vulnerable populations prepare for emergencies.

Sidebar 9-2.

Strategies for Helping Vulnerable Populations Help Themselves

Organizations can take a number of approaches to help vulnerable populations better weather an emergency. For example, in preparation for hurricane season, one Florida hospital used its case management program. The hospital worked with patients to make sure they registered with the American Red Cross or medical shelters in their neighborhoods, encouraged them to keep enough medications to care for themselves, and provided education about stocking up on supplies such as food, water, and batteries to sustain themselves during an emergency. Case managers would then contact their patients after the storms hit to determine if they had urgent medical needs.[1]

To help patients during emergencies, organizations might wish to consider providing the following materials to patients:

- A summary of their care plan, including diagnoses, allergies, medications, and past and current treatments (patients should be encouraged to carry the care plan summaries at all times)
- Copies of important documents, such as pathology reports for cancer patients
- The most recent diagnostic imaging reports

The information should be updated regularly, and patients should be encouraged to keep information in a handy, yet secure location in the event of an emergency.

References

1. Hospital helps chronically ill prepare for disaster. *Hosp Case Manag*, Aug. 1, 2007. http://0-find.galegroup.com.lrc.cod.edu:80/itx/start.do?prodID=HRCA (accessed Sep. 18, 2007).

Other Needs

The clinical and support activities standard also calls for hospitals and long term care organizations to plan for the personal hygiene and sanitation needs of patients, as well as for the mental health service needs of patients. These issues are basic to providing adequate care during an emergency, but are now spelled out explicitly in the standards.

Personal hygiene and sanitation needs have become apparent during recent disasters, such as the lack of working toilets for patients and staff during Hurricane Katrina.[5] To address these concerns, organizations should identify all of the usual activities or items that are considered essential, such as hand washing, showering, or working toilets. Then contingency plans can be made (for example, by securing portable toilets or by the general use of bedpans with specific procedures for appropriate disposal of the waste).

In addition to physical health, organizations facing emergency conditions must also consider the mental health of patients. During the emergency, organizations should consider the immediate mental health needs of those in the hospital or long term care facility. This includes a needs assessment, psychological first aid, crisis intervention, behavioral health care consultation, referrals, and so forth. Organizations can prepare for these needs by engaging in disaster behavioral health care planning and networking, specialized training initiatives for key staff, and community collaboration. During the transition to recovery from the emergency, organizations should plan for supportive counseling needs, screenings and referrals, support groups, and public education.

Mortuary Services

The standard related to managing clinical and support activities also now calls for organizations to plan for mortuary services. This reflects the fact that an emergency might produce

BE PREPARED TIP

Keep a Mortuary List

Organizations should maintain a current list of mortuaries, morgues, and other facilities that handle the dead, as well as emergency morgues.

unusual numbers of dead patients. Organizations can address this issue by collaborating with local and state coroner's offices, as well as with private mortuaries and EMS, to determine capacity and emergency plans. Community emergency preparedness typically includes plans for mortuary services, including aspects such as transportation, facilities, victim identification, necessary supplies, sanitation, disposal of remains, and other related services. Organizations should know and understand these plans, as well as make appropriate contingency plans if the community is unable to support health care organizations during an emergency. Other issues to consider related to mortuary services include supplies such as body bags, tags, and additional staff who might be necessary to process or transport fatalities.[6]

Documenting and Tracking Clinical Information

Accurate information about a patient's clinical care is the final aspect of this standard. Documenting and tracking clinical information can be particularly challenging during an emergency when, for example, there might be an influx of patients who are rapidly being triaged. Limited resources, disruptions to utilities or communication, and a host of other issues that arise during an emergency add to the complexity. Organizations could address these issues in a number of ways, such as using triage tags to identify the patient, patient condition, assessment, medications, and so forth. Documenting and tracking might also be accomplished by using a paper medical record, or a special abbreviated form of the record that has been created for emergency situations. Organizations that use wireless handheld devices such as personal digital assistants might also wish to use these (if wireless communication is possible) because of their portability, ease of use, and information-sharing capabilities. Whatever the emergency, documenting and tracking a patient's clinical information is crucial to providing safe care.

When approaching this issue, organizations can consider the following questions[7]:

- Does the organization have a method, along with the paper forms and other supplies, for recording medical information when patient volume or other conditions do not permit the use of computerized systems?
- Are tracking forms and other tools readily available in the ED that permit manual tracking of patients?
- Are tracking forms and other tools readily available in the incident command center that permit manual tracking of patients?
- Does the organization have a plan to record information that was gathered under emergency circumstances into computer systems when conditions permit?

Coordinating with the Media

The media can play a role in efforts related to clinical and support activities. For example, keeping the media abreast of an organization's care capabilities during an emergency helps to inform the public about where to seek treatment that will meet their needs. For example, the media can help get the word out about where victims with nonurgent medical needs can receive care. Organizations can also work with the media to get information out to patients who have special needs, such as those with chronic conditions.

Case Example: Caring for Residents During a Catastrophe

Residents of long term care facilities are among the frailest of the frail and the sickest of the sick. In many cases, the long term care facility is their home, and if it must be evacuated in an emergency, most of the residents would have nowhere else to go. In other words, long term care residents are completely dependent on the organization to maintain them in a site where they can be cared for.

Hurricanes and floods in the Gulf Coast and the possibility of pandemic influenza highlight the need for emergency planning in all health care organizations, especially those that focus on long term care. The vulnerability of residents is just one of several ways in which long term care organizations are different from hospitals and other health care organizations during an emergency.

Federal and state regulators require every long term care organization to prepare for emergencies. The Joint Commission's emergency management standards also require organizations to develop detailed plans that take into account different emergencies and contingencies, and organizations must review and revise these plans regularly.

Staffing

In addition to the vulnerability and dependence of their residents, another area in which long term care organizations differ from hospitals in their emergency planning efforts is staffing. According to Janice Zalen, senior director, Special Programs, American Health Care Association (AHCA), the turnover in leadership and staff at long term care organizations is often higher than at other kinds of organizations, with fewer physicians and nurses and many more certified nursing assistants (CNAs). "That can mean a different level of skill and less training for staff," says Zalen. In some cases, that could translate into personnel who might be less prepared to deal with the clinical and environmental challenges of emergency management.

One problem that emerged during the 2005 hurricanes in the Gulf Coast region is that long term care personnel were blocked in their attempts to get to work. Like almost everyone else in that region, they were sidelined by a shortage of gasoline when generators were flooded and there was no power to pump fuel out of underground storage tanks at gas stations. "Hospital personnel could use their [identification] badges to get what little fuel there was," Zalen recalls, "but not our nursing assistants." AHCA recommended that nursing facilities give CNAs a letter to show to gas stations, but some CNAs were still turned away because many of those facility names sound more like gated communities or resorts than nursing homes.

Evacuation and Special Clinical Needs

The process of evacuation when the long term care facility can no longer support adequate care, treatment, and services can be even more challenging than evacuating a hospital. Because of the time and work associated with moving residents of a nursing home, facilities need to start evacuations sooner rather than later, says Zalen. "Many residents have special needs, such as receiving dialysis or being on ventilators. And it can take a long time to get them onto buses and ambulances," she says. But if the facility evacuates its residents and the emergency *doesn't* strike, the federal government won't reimburse the facility for the cost of evacuation. This could cost the facility's management as much as $150,000.

Zalen cites a case in which a nursing home in the Florida Keys was right in the projected path of a storm. Residents were evacuated north to Orlando. At the last minute, the hurricane turned aside without striking the Keys, but a tornado did strike Orlando.

(continued)

Case Example: Caring for Residents During a Catastrophe, *continued*

Dementia

Arguably the chief factor that differentiates residents of long term care organizations from hospital patients is the prevalence of dementia among residents. It is estimated that approximately half of all nursing home residents have Alzheimer's disease or a related disorder.[1] Due to their loss of cognitive ability, residents with dementia will require extra help and consideration when an emergency plan is implemented.

Nursing home residents might not be able to adequately feed or hydrate themselves and will also need special assistance with toileting or other hygiene needs during an emergency and its aftermath. Residents with dementia might not be able to follow or remember instructions about hand washing, wearing a protective face mask, not putting things in their mouths, staying in a particular area, or other matters that involve individual follow-through and accountability.

Residents with dementia could become disoriented and pose a danger to themselves or others if they are not in their usual secure environment. They are susceptible to agitation, frustration, and even catastrophic reactions during a crisis situation, and they have a reduced ability to tolerate changes in their environment.

Another hazard among residents with dementia is wandering, which means aimless or purposeful activity that causes a social problem—getting lost, leaving a safe environment, or intruding in inappropriate places. The risk for wandering increases when residents become upset or agitated or when they face stressful situations.

Residents who have dementia are particularly susceptible to a catastrophic reaction, which can occur when a situation overloads the mental ability of the person with dementia to act rationally. The person then has an exaggerated response to the situation and can strike out, scream, make unreasonable accusations, or become highly agitated or emotional. In the changes and chaos of an emergency or an evacuation, residents are more likely to undergo a catastrophic reaction to a new situation or a changed environment.

These manifestations of dementia become even more difficult for overburdened staff members to cope with during an emergency.

Updating the Plan

Although long term care organizations must test emergency operations plans twice a year, some organizations learn new information through unfortunate real-life experiences. Kaleida Health in Buffalo, New York, has four long term care facilities. A fire in a service area at one of the facilities in 2005 was caught early, before it could threaten any of the 160 residents. The focus was on the residents, but the organization learned about staff safety in the process.

After firefighters left, staff members worked to quickly get things back to normal for residents. Because the staff members worked on the cleanup process without respiratory protection, many staff inhaled soot and later began experiencing problems with their breathing. The organization began reviewing its emergency plan so that it could add provisions that require staff protection in case of a fire or other emergency.

Reference

1. Alzheimer's Association: *2008 Alzheimer's Disease Facts and Figures.* 2008. http://www.alz.org/national/documents/report_alzfactsfigures2008.pdf (accessed Mar. 23, 2006).

Source: Reprinted from Joint Commission Resources: Emergency management in long term care. *Environment of Care News* 9:9, Sep. 2006.

Case Example: Preparing for a Pediatric Mass Casualty

When Liberty Hospital in Liberty, Missouri, developed a disaster plan, staff made certain to incorporate steps for dealing with pediatric patients. On May 9, 2005, that plan was put to the test when a school bus lost control while going through an intersection and collided with two passenger vehicles. Minutes after the crash, Liberty got a call describing the events and telling staff to activate the disaster plan. At least 40 to 50 children were injured, and many of them would be brought to Liberty Hospital.

Staff leaped into action:

- The emergency department (ED) clinical director assumed the role of incident commander, and the assistant ED nurse manager became the treatment area's director.
- Two ED nurses were assigned to the two incoming patients that emergency medical services (EMS) had triaged as critical, and another ED nurse stayed at the ambulance entrance to give room assignments to EMS crews bringing in patients.
- The ED had just one pediatric crash cart, so the special procedures and pediatrics unit sent down their carts as well.
- Three critical care rooms with crash carts were set up, and a pharmacist was made available for each one.

In less than 10 minutes, the disaster plan was under way, and the hospital was ready to receive and treat a large volume of pediatric patients. Moments later, the first injured children began to arrive.

Because the children were on a school bus and not with their parents, hospital staff knew that a flood of family members could be expected to arrive soon after the patients. To help with the flow of people, staff placed identification bands on the wrists of those parents who had already been matched up with their children. In addition, the family waiting area was moved a short distance away from the ED, thus relieving some of the congestion in the main ED areas. Liberty also had enough nurses come to the ED from other areas of the hospital that it was able to assign at least one staff person to stay with each child throughout his or her treatment, which eased a lot of the anxiety of the patients and their families.

A total of 29 crash victims—27 children and 2 adults—were treated in the Liberty ED, and 21 of them arrived by ambulance within the first hour. Six of those patients were admitted, 1 went to the operating room, and 5 were transferred to a nearby children's hospital.

Other than a few minor glitches, the disaster plan was implemented as well as Liberty staff could have hoped, and the hospital was commended by the local EMS companies, other facilities, and the community for its successful efforts that day.

Source: Reprinted from Behney A., Breit M., Phillips C.: Pediatric mass casualty: Are you ready? *J Emerg Nurs* 32:341–245, Jun. 2006, with permission from the Emergency Nurses Association.

Case Example: Emergency Preparation for Pediatric Patients

Children are at higher risk than adults in emergency situations. They have smaller blood and fluid reserves than adults, and thus their conditions can deteriorate more rapidly. Their faster breathing patterns and thinner skin put them at increased risk of harm due to exposure to biological or chemical agents. Their immature motor and cognitive skills can slow them in circumstances calling for quick action.

"Because early emergency medical services (EMS) systems were developed in the late 1960s and were based on techniques learned during past war efforts, they tended to focus on adults," says Mark Cichon, D.O., principal investigator, Emergency Medical Services for Children (EMSC), Loyola University Health System, Maywood, Illinois. "By the 1970s and early 1980s we began to recognize that medical professionals out in the field and even in hospitals were not fully equipped with the necessary tools and training to address the unique medical needs of children. Even though much has been accomplished to better address pediatric emergency care needs, there is still more that can be done."

The EMSC program is a national initiative dedicated to improving emergency care for pediatric patients. Designed to reduce child and youth disability and death due to severe illness and injury, it is the only federal program that focuses specifically on improving the quality of children's emergency care. All states, U.S. territories, and the District of Columbia have received federal funding to support EMSC programs. Because each state is different and might have different pediatric needs and priorities, each is encouraged to sketch out its own goals and objectives within a framework defined by the national EMSC program. That framework focuses on programming that improves existing EMS systems as well as develops and evaluates improved procedures and protocols for treating children. Currently, only state governments and accredited schools of medicine are eligible to receive EMSC grants.

The Web site of the national EMSC program, at http://www.ems-c.org, provides a list of each state's EMSC coordinator/contact. In Illinois, EMSC is a collaborative program between the Illinois Department of Public Health and Loyola University Health System. As manager of the Illinois EMSC program, Evelyn Lyons coordinates a collective effort that since 1994 has worked to ensure that health care providers and health care facilities in Illinois are prepared to meet the emergency care needs of children. Beginning in 1998, the Illinois Department of Public Health began formally recognizing Illinois hospitals for their emergency department (ED) pediatric preparedness through the EMSC Pediatric Facility Recognition process. "This is a voluntary process in which hospitals strive to meet specific criteria ensuring that they have appropriately trained personnel and the proper resources and capabilities to effectively treat a critically ill or injured child," says Lyons.

Supported by a committee made up of representatives from other key state agencies and professional organizations, the Illinois EMSC has established three levels of participation, based on varying levels of criteria. All Illinois hospitals are encouraged to gain recognition as one of the following:

- Standby Emergency Department Approved for Pediatrics (SEDAP)—This level is typically associated with a smaller hospital that has policies, training, and other resources in place to initially manage and stabilize a child. In addition, this level requires the ability to refer patients to more thoroughly equipped pediatric facilities, when appropriate.
- Emergency Department Approved for Pediatrics (EDAP)—A comprehensive facility including 24-hour physician coverage that might admit pediatric patients but might not have pediatric intensive care and other pediatric inpatient services needed in certain circumstances.
- Pediatric Critical Care Center (PCCC)—A facility with a more comprehensive range of pediatric services that goes beyond the ED and includes a pediatric intensive care unit and other pediatric specialty services.

(continued)

Case Example: Emergency Preparation for Pediatric Patients, *continued*

EMSC Pediatric Facility Recognition is an initial step in preparing for pediatric disaster and terrorist events. Through consultations, site visits, and resource sharing, the EMSC program assists Illinois health care organizations in achieving these levels of recognition.

Complementing Joint Commission standards on emergency management, the Illinois EMSC has also developed a guideline for hospitals to assist in identifying key pediatric considerations to integrate into their overall disaster plans. Although this is a comprehensive undertaking, there are some tips health care organizations should consider as they approach the steps of this important process.

- **Prepare for unexpected patients.** For health care organizations preparing for the possibility of an emergency intake, the current awareness of terrorist activity should raise new questions about readiness to deal with a heavy volume of admissions. This includes conducting population-specific assessments, according to Lyons. "Conduct an internal assessment of how 'pediatric prepared' your facility is. In a mass-casualty incident, it is likely that the resources to assist children will be scarce. Staff inexperience with pediatric critical injury and illness will result in an inadequate surge capacity," she says. "Organizations must predetermine whether they have an adequate number of staff who are trained in pediatric emergency care. In addition, this assessment must include an evaluation of on-site pediatric-specific equipment, as well as assure that there are mechanisms in place to quickly secure additional pediatric supplies." In responding to an actual incident, health care facilities should find out as quickly as possible the potential number of pediatric victims they can expect in order to begin preparations to manage the care of children. As facilities work to develop strategies to increase their surge capacity, they need to ensure that these strategies are consistent with their EMS regional disaster plan.
- **Assess your community's risk.** A health care organization should assess specific threats unique to the physical structure, the campus, and the geographic environment of its facility through a hazard vulnerability analysis (HVA), as required by the standard discussed in Chapter 2. In performing an HVA, a health care organization can identify areas where children regularly convene—such as schools, parks, and summer camps—and determine what types of hazards have a high, medium, or low probability of occurring.
- **Conduct and evaluate pediatric drills.** The EMSC program stresses the importance of including a sufficient proportion of pediatric victims and child-related scenarios in all plans to test the emergency operations plan (as also required by Joint Commission standards) and tabletop exercises, as well as conducting drills that exclusively involve pediatric victims, to test the capacity of an organization's system to handle pediatric patients. "Ongoing evaluation of your pediatric emergency care capabilities is key," says Lyons. "In the EMSC Pediatric Facility Recognition process, organizations at all levels of participation are required to have a continuous quality improvement (CQI) liaison, a staff member whose job it is to ensure the pediatric quality improvement process. [He or she] evaluates pediatric care within their emergency department and also works with other hospital CQI liaisons within their EMS region to address pediatric issues more broadly throughout their region."
- **Reach out to other agencies.** A vital aspect of emergency preparation involves nurturing relationships with local law enforcement agencies, fire departments, children's hospitals, public health services, and others. Organizations should be aware of and collaborate with local, state, and regional emergency response teams.
- **Prepare staff to be specially equipped.** "EMS is still a relatively young field, and the integration of a pediatrics focus is still evolving, so ongoing staff training and education is essential to an organization's emergency preparation efforts," says Lyons.

Source: Adapted from Joint Commission Resources: Emergency preparation for special populations, part 1: Pediatrics. *Environment of Care News* 8:12, Dec. 2005.

For Additional Assistance

- JumpSTART Pediatric MCI Triage Tool: http://www.jumpstarttriage.com/JumpSTART_and_MCI_Triage.php
- New York City Department of Health and Mental Hygiene—Pediatric Disaster Toolkit: Hospital Guidelines for Pediatrics During Disasters: http://www.nyc.gov/html/doh/html/bhpp/bhpp-focus-ped-toolkit.shtml
- American Academy of Pediatrics, Children, Terrorism & Disaster Toolkit: http://www.aap.org/terrorism/index.html
- Pennsylvania Department of Health: Special Populations Emergency Preparedness Planning: http://www.dsf.health.state.pa.us/health/cwp/view.asp?a=333&q=233957
- Disability Preparedness Center: http://www.disabilitypreparedness.org
- Substance Abuse and Mental Health Services Administration's Disaster Technical Assistance Center: http://www.mentalhealth.samhsa.gov/dtac
- Disaster Mortuary Operational Response Teams: http://www.dmort.org/

References

1. Dewan S., Baker A.: Owners of nursing home charged in deaths of 34. *New York Times,* Sep. 14, 2005. http://www.nytimes.com/2005/09/14/national/nationalspecial/14storm.html (accessed Nov. 1, 2007).
2. Markenson D., Redlener I.: Pediatric terrorism preparedness national guidelines and recommendations: Findings of an evidence-based consensus process. *Biosecur Bioterror* 4:301–319, 2004.
3. American Academy of Pediatrics Committee on Pediatric Emergency Medicine, Committee on Medical Liability, and Task Force on Terrorism: Policy statement: The pediatrician and disaster preparedness. *Pediatrics* 117, Feb. 2006. http://aappolicy.aappublications.org/cgi/content/full/pediatrics;117/2/560 (accessed Nov. 13, 2007).
4. Joint Commission Resources: Emergency preparation for special populations, part 2: Geriatric and special needs. *Environment of Care News* 9:4, Apr. 2006.
5. Joint Commission Resources: 10 lessons from escalating disasters. *Environment of Care News* 9:2, Feb. 2006.
6. Garner A. Documentation and tagging of casualties in multiple casualty incidents. *Emergency Medicine* 15(5–6):475–479, 2003.
7. American Health Lawyers Association: *Emergency Preparedness, Response & Recovery Checklist: Beyond the Emergency Management Plan.* Washington, DC: American Health Lawyers Association, 2004.

Chapter 10

Testing the Emergency Operations Plan

Exercises, formerly referred to by The Joint Commission as drills, are an integral element of an effective emergency operations plan (EOP). Periodically testing the plan enables organizations to assess the plan's appropriateness and adequacy and the effectiveness of logistics, human resources, training, policies, procedures, and protocols. The basic goal is to assess preparedness capabilities and performance when systems are stressed during an actual emergency. If those tests sufficiently stress the organization's processes, the exercise reveals the strengths and weaknesses of the plan and leads to improvements.

This chapter discusses the use of regular, planned exercises to help troubleshoot weaknesses in EOPs and includes a number of checklists, strategies, tools, and case examples that health care organizations can use to help ensure that their EOPs are as complete as possible. *See* Sidebar 10-1 (page 132) for the Joint Commission's requirements related to testing the EOP.

Testing EOPs

The standard is designed to assist health care organizations to test their EOP, identify deficiencies, and take corrective actions to continuously improve the effectiveness of their EOP. Only a thorough and objective evaluation of performance during an emergency management event or planned exercise will demonstrate how effective the organization's planning efforts have been.

Periodic testing of an EOP enables organizations to assess the plan's appropriateness and adequacy, as well as the effectiveness of logistics, human resources, training, policies, procedures, and protocols. Exercises should stress the limits of the organization's emergency management system. The goal of this testing is to assess the organization's preparedness capabilities and performance when systems are stressed during an actual emergency.

Exercises should be developed using plausible scenarios that are realistic and relevant to the organizations. Events should be based on each organization's hazard vulnerability analysis (HVA). Exercises should also validate the effectiveness of the plan and identify opportunities to improve.

It is important to communicate the strengths and weaknesses of the performance revealed by the exercise to all levels of the organization, including administration, clinical staff, governing body, and those responsible for managing the patient safety program. Sidebar 10-2 (page 133) examines research by the Agency for Healthcare Research and Quality (AHRQ) regarding lessons learned during exercises.

Conducting Exercises

Organizations are expected to test their EOP twice a year, either in response to an actual emergency or in a planned exercise. The timing of the two exercises is left up to each

Be Prepared Tip

Staying Current

Emergency management exercises should be based on the high-priority hazard identified in an organization's hazard vulnerability analysis (HVA); however, organizations should not consider the HVA to be a static document. Just as that document should be revised regularly to reflect the current threats an organization faces, the types of exercises conducted should also change according to the most current kinds of hazards that could affect the organization.

Sidebar 10-1.

Applicable Emergency Management Standard

The organization regularly tests the emergency operations plan.

This standard requires the following:

Number and Types of Exercises

- The organization tests its emergency operations plan twice a year, either in response to an actual emergency or in a planned exercise. Note that staff in freestanding buildings classified as a business occupancy (as defined by the *Life Safety Code*®*) that does not offer emergency services and is not community-designated as a disaster-receiving station need to conduct only one emergency preparedness exercise annually. Also note that tabletop sessions, though useful, are not acceptable substitutes for exercises.
- In the cases of critical access hospitals and long term care institutions, organizations that offer emergency services or are community-designated disaster receiving stations conduct at least one exercise a year that includes an influx of actual or simulated patients.
- At least one exercise a year is escalated to evaluate how effectively the organization performs when it cannot be supported by the local community. Note that tabletop sessions are acceptable in meeting the community portion of this exercise.

Organizations that have a defined role in the communitywide emergency management program participate in at least one communitywide exercise a year. *Communitywide* may range from a contiguous geographic area served by the same health care providers to a large borough, town, city, or region. Also note that the exercises for the aforementioned requirements may be conducted separately or simultaneously. And again, tabletop sessions are acceptable in meeting the community portion of this exercise.

Scope of Exercises

- Planned exercise scenarios are realistic and related to the priority emergencies identified in the organization's hazard vulnerability analysis.
- During planned exercises, an individual whose sole responsibility is to monitor performance (and who is knowledgeable in the goals and expectations of the exercise) documents opportunities for improvement. (This individual may be a staff member of the organization who is not participating in the exercise.)
- During planned exercises, the organization monitors, at a minimum, the following six critical areas:
  1. Communication, including the effectiveness of communication both within the organization as well as with response entities outside of the organization, such as local government leadership, police, fire, public health, and other health care organizations within the community
  2. Resources and assets, including responders, equipment, supplies, personal protective equipment, and transportation
  3. Safety and security
  4. Staff roles and responsibilities
  5. Utilities management
  6. Patient clinical and support activities
- Exercises are critiqued to identify deficiencies and opportunities for improvement based on monitoring activities and observations during the exercise.
- Completed exercises are critiqued through a multidisciplinary process that includes administration and clinical steps. In the cases of critical access hospitals and long term care organizations, this includes physicians and support staff.
- The organization modifies its emergency operations plan in response to critiques of exercises.
- Planned exercises evaluate the effectiveness of improvements that were made in response to critiques of the previous exercise. Note that when improvements require substantive resources that cannot be accomplished by the next planned exercise, interim improvements must be put in place until final resolution.
- The strengths and weaknesses identified during exercises are communicated to the mutlidisciplinary improvement team responsible for monitoring environment-of-care issues.

* *Life Safety Code* is a registered trademark of the National Fire Protection Association, Quincy, MA.

Sidebar 10-2.

Lessons Learned in Disaster Drills

To find out more about what organizations are learning from their disaster drills, the Agency for Healthcare Research and Quality conducted a review of the current literature. Because the drills varied in terms of targeted staff, learning objectives, identified outcomes, and evaluation methods, it was difficult to draw definitive conclusions about the most effective approaches for training hospital staff to respond to a disaster. However, researchers uncovered some interesting lessons:

- Internal and external communications were key to effective disaster response.
- Having a well-defined incident command center reduced confusion.
- Conducting conference calls was an inefficient way to manage disaster response.
- Having accurate phone numbers for key players was vital, and regular updating was necessary.
- Conducting disaster drills appeared to be an effective way to improve clinicians' knowledge of hospital disaster procedures.
- Computer simulation might be an economical method to educate key hospital decision makers and improve hospital disaster preparedness before implementation to a full-scale drill.
- A tabletop exercise can help motivate hospital staff to learn more about disaster preparedness and can help teach staff about aspects of disaster-related patient care in a way that simulates the practice setting.
- Conducting a regional exercise involving top government officials can help increase awareness of the need for better disaster-response planning.
- Video demonstrations might be an inexpensive, convenient way to educate a large number of staff about disaster procedures and equipment use in a short time.

Source: Agency for Healthcare Research and Quality (AHRQ): *Training of Hospital Staff to Respond to a Mass Casualty Incident.* Rockville, MD: AHRQ, Apr. 2004.

Be Prepared Tip

Injecting "Reality"

To inject as much "reality" into the exercise as possible, consider the exercise's duration, complexity, and resource utilization when planning it. For example, organizations might want to conduct an exercise in the evening or at night when there are fewer staff members working. If the exercise occurs during off-peak hours, then off-peak staffing should respond. The organization cannot assume that it will be able to get its day-shift staff to return to work that evening.

organization. For long term care organizations and critical access hospitals that offer emergency services or are community-designated disaster receiving stations, at least one exercise a year must include an influx of actual or simulated patients. Organizations can determine the particular emergency scenario for the influx of volunteers or simulated patients, as well as the escalating exercise.

Volunteers are just that—usually community members who have been recruited to represent emergency victims. Simulated patients, sometimes known as "paper patients," are usually cards with symptoms written on them. If simulated care recipients are used, they must be triaged, put on gurneys or in wheelchairs, and transported through the system as if they were actually receiving care at the organization. Regardless of whether volunteers or simulated patients are used, organizations should apply a realistic time line, and utilization of the six critical areas of emergency management should mirror a real event.

Because mass-casualty events can generate hundreds or thousands of victims, an exercise should reflect that scenario and simulate the challenges that accompany a surge of individuals seeking care. Among those questions are, How would the organization triage hundreds of patients at one time? Where would the organization isolate or decontaminate them if either were necessary? Does the organization have enough pharmaceuticals to treat them? Does it have enough food and water to feed them?

BE PREPARED TIP

Tabletop Exercises

Tabletop sessions, though useful, are not acceptable substitutes for the twice-a-year exercises required by the standard. Tabletop sessions *are* acceptable in meeting the community portion of the required escalation exercise and are useful to gather input on planning and designing emergency management procedures.

The second required drill per year may be another external emergency. However, it is recommended that organizations use the opportunity to test some portion of the internal EOP. For example, weather emergencies or utility failures might be the focus of the exercise. The checklist contained in Table 10-1 (at right) offers a starting point for organizations seeking to test an EOP.

Escalating the Exercise

As previously mentioned, organizations are required to conduct at least one exercise a year that is escalated so that the organization can determine how it will cope without the support of the local community. Conducting exercises involving multiple elements of an emergency at one time, such as a large influx of patients and a simultaneous loss of power, makes the drill more realistic. For example, a hurricane could cause an organization to lose power for two weeks, could contaminate its water supply, could prevent some staff members from arriving at the facility due to flooded roads, and could also prevent food supplies from reaching the organization. The events of September 11, 2001, when the World Trade Center towers collapsed, also show how emergencies can escalate. On that day, there were plane crashes, major fires, two building collapses, mass casualties, a public health emergency, and loss of utilities.

Unless the exercise stresses the system, it will not provide insight into strengths and weaknesses. To accomplish this, the exercise should not only require using additional supplies and equipment, but it should also drain on-hand inventory to test organization processes for obtaining more equipment, medical supplies, pharmaceuticals, food, water, linens, and so forth. Exercises should push participants to explore existing agreements with suppliers and to investigate new ones. For example, the organization might have a designated individual call vendors to explain that an exercise is in progress and to ask how long it would take to deliver the supplies. This tests the ability to reach suppliers and see how quickly they can deliver the needed supplies and equipment.

Table 10-1. Checklist for Conducting Exercises

- ❑ Does the organization conduct regular exercises?
- ❑ Do the exercises ensure that all key participants are familiar with the contents of the emergency operations plan?
- ❑ Are specific aspects of the plan measured?
- ❑ Is a formal "after-action" critique performed, with results distributed to all key individuals and participating groups?

Source: Adapted from Association for Professionals in Infection Control and Epidemiology. Center for the Study of Bioterrorism and Emerging Infections: *Mass-Casualty Disaster Plan Checklist: A Template for Healthcare Facilities.* http://bioterrorism.slu.edu/bt/quick/disasterplan.pdf (accessed Mar. 10, 2008).

The exercise should also push staffing to its limits. A designated individual on each unit should make calls to see which staff members can report to work and how long it will take them to get there. This will ensure that call lists are current. If the telephones are not working, the organization must use its communications backup systems to contact staff. If staff members are unable to get to the organization because of inclement weather, then the organization should consider its transportation options for picking them up. If staff members will not report to work because of fears of contamination or other related fears of personal safety, then the organization should practice during its exercise how to obtain additional staff, such as volunteers or staff from other organizations. If staff members cannot be present because they are caring for their families, the organization should consider including in an exercise the establishment of an area as a shelter for the staff's family members.

Other Considerations

Exercises are integral to the process of troubleshooting weaknesses in EOPs. When setting up an EOP exercise, organizations should carefully decide on its components. It is also important to note that the standard now requires organizations

Sidebar 10-3.
Take Disaster Drills Seriously

Beyond fulfilling the requirements of the standard, it is important for everyone in an organization to understand that effective exercises must be given serious and comprehensive attention. Drill every aspect of the emergency operations plan, including the following:
- Testing and retesting all equipment that will be used during an emergency (for example, communication backups, emergency generator, staff notifications, and so forth)
- Involving community agencies
- Deploying the clinical staff
- Setting up the incident command center
- Evacuating and transporting the patient population
- Requesting and receiving emergency supplies and equipment from other organizations
- Managing safety and security during the simulated emergency

to monitor the six critical areas of emergency management (communication, resources and assets, safety and security, staff roles and responsibilities, utilities management, and patient clinical and support activities) during planned exercises.

Organizations can consider the following questions to make the exercises meaningful[1]:
- What will the emergency be? This should be as specific as possible to offer the most realistic test of the plan. For example, a mock disaster involving bioterrorism should be specific, as clinical treatments vary, depending on the problem.
- Which departments in the organization will be involved? For example, it makes sense to go beyond the emergency department (ED) in a hospital or clinical care areas in a nursing home to reach into other areas that would be called upon during an emergency. For example, will pharmacy or the laboratory be included?
- Will the exercise run across multiple shifts?
- How can the exercise be conducted without disrupting normal care provided?
- How will patients and the community be made aware of the exercise so that it is not mistaken for a real crisis?
- How can the exercise be made scalable? In other words, how can the exercise be escalated or contracted?
- What supplies and equipment will be included in the exercise?
- How will communication, including the effectiveness of communication both within the organization and with those in the community, be maintained and monitored?
- What provisions will need to be made for safety and security, both as part of the planned exercise and to maintain normal operations?

The organization must also determine how and when the exercise will end: Will it be completed at a certain time of day or when a particular outcome is achieved? Either way, the end of the exercise should be specific and tightly controlled, with a detailed plan for returning to normal activity in a way that minimizes confusion and disorder and ensures that useful information is not lost in the shuffle. Often, exercises are concluded too early. It is not until systems break down that real learning occurs. Escalating the exercise, as now required, shows organizations how "drilling to failure" is the best means to identify systems and processes that are at risk.

Organizations might also wish to consider conducting exercises for emergencies that extend past a few hours or days. Staff might be able to respond to an immediate emergency, but what happens beyond a few days, weeks, or even months as was the case with the 2003 severe acute respiratory syndrome (SARS) epidemic in Toronto? How will the organization continue to maintain a sufficient number and mix of staff over time? How will it rotate staff? How will staff members balance their professional responsibilities with their personal needs to take care of family members or deal with losing their home due to natural disasters? Sidebar 10-3 (above) provides a list of issues to consider when testing the EOP.

Communitywide Exercises
The standard regarding EOP testing also requires participation in at least one communitywide emergency management exercise a year. *Communitywide* might range from a contiguous geographic area served by the same health care providers to a large borough, town, city, or region. The drill should be rele-

vant to potential threats identified in the HVA and should assess the communication, coordination, and effectiveness of both the organization's and the community's command structures. All major emergency response participants should be included. Among them are the health care organization(s), local leaders, public health authorities, emergency medical services, fire department, police department, local businesses, and volunteer patients. Alternative care sites should be included because testing increases communitywide awareness of the existence, location, strengths, and challenges of such facilities. It also encourages face-to-face interactions so that responders become familiar with one another.

BE PREPARED TIP

Testing Personal Protective Equipment

When conducting an exercise, hospitals should require health care workers to put on and remove personal protective equipment. This will enable health care workers to experience conditions that simulate some of the physical and mental challenges of conducting patient care tasks while wearing biosuits. The ability of workers to don and remove isolation garments without contaminating themselves should also be tested.

Monitoring the Six Critical Areas

One of the new requirements related to the standard is carefully monitoring the six critical areas of emergency management—communication, resources and assets, safety and security, staff responsibilities, utilities management, and patient clinical and support activities. If, during an emergency or a planned exercise, an organization cannot handle one or more of these critical areas—because of the nature of the emergency and situation—the organization might need to consider evacuating to another location. Ideally, an organization should be able to manage these six areas during an emergency, but if it cannot, it is important to identify weaknesses and improvement opportunities through exercises. Identifying those weaknesses and understanding what improvements have been made will help organizations ensure that they do not wait until it is too late to evacuate.

Next Steps

Following an emergency and implementation of the EOP, health care organizations should conduct a technical debriefing or evaluation. Organization performance must be monitored during planned exercises by an individual whose sole responsibility is to do just that. This individual can get the evaluation process started. The evaluation should be a candid, closed-door meeting that analyzes the organization's effectiveness in dealing with the emergency. Key staff members from all departments should be included. Questions for the sessions include, among others: Did the plan function the way it should have? What failed? What worked? How many patients were treated? What categories of patients were treated? How many discharges, admissions, deaths, and transfers occurred? How were departments staffed? Was staffing appropriate? Was equipment provided as needed? How might communications systems have been improved? Were other utility systems adequate, and if not, how might they be improved?

There are two ways to think about the timing of critiques, and both approaches have merit. One method is to give managers and supervisors at least two days' advance notice of any post-emergency debriefing or evaluation. This helps ensure that they can obtain staff input prior to the meeting. Another approach is to schedule the critique immediately following the exercise because individuals' memories of what happened can fade quickly. Ask what worked well and what did not, and decide what to do about the latter. In either approach, it is important to consider what can be done about areas for improvement or else the organization does not benefit from the full value of the exercise. Table 10-2 (page 137) provides a checklist that could be used for evaluating exercises through a group debriefing.

It is also important, though, that the monitoring of the exercises and subsequent analysis focus on measurable objectives. EOPs and their implementation lack meaning without performance measures, which offer a way to measure whether and how well the organization implemented its plans. Agreeing on what constitutes success and identifying performance measures during the emergency management planning stages (discussed in Chapters 2 and 3) will help determine the exercise's effectiveness and contribute to improved future performance. For example, an acute care hospital conducting a bioterrorist exercise involving smallpox identified four objectives[2]:

- Discuss the use of smallpox as a biological weapon.
- Demonstrate the disease's epidemic potential.
- Identify staffing impact.
- Discuss the process of networking with local, state, and federal agencies.

Table 10-2. Group Debriefing Checklist

This checklist is based on the Agency for Healthcare Research and Quality's module-based approach for evaluating disaster exercises. The following questions are relevant to every zone involved in the exercise. When responding to the questions, the debriefing participants should state their zone.

- ❑ Did you feel you were notified of the disaster in a timely fashion?
- ❑ Did the incident command center work effectively?
- ❑ Did any zone receive incorrect information from the incident command center? If not correct, what specifics do you recall about incorrect information?
- ❑ Was the information from the incident command center received by other zones in a timely way? Did the hospital experience problems with information flow?
- ❑ Were memorandums of understanding with outside agencies (such as police) activated? Were they functional?
- ❑ Did nurses and physicians respond quickly to the disaster call?
- ❑ Was the zone set up when the first mock victim arrived?
- ❑ Was security in place before the first mock victim arrived?
- ❑ Did people have a good understanding of their roles, as defined in the disaster plan?
- ❑ Did the decontamination system work effectively?
- ❑ Did you have any problems with the decontamination equipment? Functioning properly? Adequate number of units? Participants used it correctly?
- ❑ Were there delays in decontamination? If so, what triggered these delays?
- ❑ Did the triage system work effectively?
- ❑ Were there delays in triage? If so, what triggered these delays?
- ❑ Did the treatment system work effectively?
- ❑ Were there delays in treatment? If so, what triggered these delays?
- ❑ Was personal protective equipment (PPE) used correctly?
- ❑ Were you able to function in the PPE?
- ❑ Were you rotated adequately when wearing the PPE?
- ❑ Was security adequate?
- ❑ Was staffing adequate?
- ❑ Were supplies adequate?
- ❑ Was the equipment adequate? If not, what equipment was not adequate (give specifics)?
- ❑ Were there problems with transporting patients?
- ❑ Were there problems with communication devices (such as equipment failure)?
- ❑ Did the hospital appear to work well with city and/or regional disaster agencies?
- ❑ Were there problems with information flow between the hospital and outside agencies? If yes, which agencies?
- ❑ Were there bottlenecks?
- ❑ Was workspace adequate?
- ❑ Did you feel you could accomplish what you were assigned to do during the exercise?
- ❑ What did you learn from participating in the exercise?
- ❑ Overall, what parts of the exercise went well?
- ❑ What could have been done differently to make the exercise run better?

Source: Adapted from Cosgrove S.E., et al.: *Group Debriefing Modules in Evaluation of Hospital Disaster Drills: A Module-Based Approach.* Agency for Healthcare Research and Quality (AHRQ), AHRQ Publication No. 04-0032. Apr. 2004. http://www.ahrq.gov/research/hospdrills (accessed Nov. 14, 2007).

Table 10-3. Checklist for Testing and Revising the Emergency Operations Plan

- ❑ The organization regularly conducts emergency exercises (either in response to an actual emergency or in planned exercises).
- ❑ Health care workers are required to don and remove personal protective equipment during exercises.
- ❑ The exercises use measurable objectives.
- ❑ The organization conducts exercises that simulate an influx of patients, using volunteers or simulated patients.
- ❑ The organization conducts communitywide practice exercises.
- ❑ The organization conducts tabletop exercises.
- ❑ The exercises address the six critical aspects of emergency management—communication, resources and assets, safety and security, staff responsibilities, utilities management, and patient clinical and support activities.
- ❑ The organization critiques its exercises to improve preparedness and response capabilities.
- ❑ External observers are recruited to critique exercises.
- ❑ The organization reviews the emergency operations plan on an annual basis and reprioritizes hazards as necessary.
- ❑ Information obtained from tests, exercises, and after-action reports is used to improve preparedness and response plans.

Be Prepared Tip

Recruit External Observers

One way to enhance objectivity during a critique is to recruit external observers. The organization should train the observers to ensure that they know what to look for. Provide them with written criteria to guide their evaluations and station them in strategic areas or zones.

Be Prepared Tip

Soliciting Input

Consider getting comments from both nonlicensed and licensed staff about the exercise's effectiveness. Also, request comments from other organizations, such as emergency medical services, that participated in the tests.

The collection and analysis of data relevant to answering such questions are key to performance improvement. EOPs and their implementation lack meaning without performance measures—a way to measure whether and how well the organization implemented its plans. A performance measure is used to determine whether a process, function, or service is actually performing according to identified expectations. During the planning stages, organization leaders must ensure that staff define appropriate performance measures. These could be related to such key areas as staff knowledge and skills, implementation of established procedures, provision of needed equipment, and so forth. The measures might address any one or more of the nine dimensions of performance—efficacy, appropriateness, availability, timeliness, effectiveness, continuity, safety, efficiency, and respect and caring. Good measures move organizations toward improvement by enabling them to evaluate the effectiveness of their emergency management plans.

Lessons learned from an evaluation of performance measurement data can then be applied to revise the plan. Whether it was an actual event or a planned exercise, it is important that the critique, corrective action plans, and other appropriate documentation be made available in a written report to those responsible for safety considerations to make sure corrective actions are carried out. Health care organizations throughout the United States are being challenged to respond and improve their readiness to respond effectively to many types of emergencies. A thorough review by each health care organization of its emergency management plan is critical, and such reviews must be regular and ongoing. The all-hazards approach to emergency management planning and implementation recommended by The Joint Commission will go a long way toward ensuring that health care organizations don't have to reinvent the wheel with each new emergency. Table 10-3 (above) provides a checklist that organizations could use as a starting point for testing and revising the EOP.

Coordinating with the Media

All local media should be contacted when an organization tests its emergency operations plan. This prevents misunderstandings about whether the event is a real emergency and provides an opportunity to share with the public how the organization strives to be ready to serve the community during a variety of emergency scenarios. Members of the media might also ask to report on the exercises, which offers a chance to test how the organization would make accommodations for the media during a real emergency.

CASE EXAMPLE:
EVALUATING A REAL-LIFE EMERGENCY

The critique of a real-life emergency in which a man drove his car through the main entrance of 700-bed St. Vincent Hospital in Indianapolis, resulting in a fire, was conducted the following week and attended by the hospital's vice president of clinical and nonclinical support services, director of facility services, manager of security services, the security team leader, director of emergency services, fire alarm technicians, director of nursing administration, and manager of health and safety, as well as personnel from the township fire department. Among the postincident changes made to the hospital's emergency management plan were retraining regarding the emergency code and the importance of implementing the disaster plan; training leadership, which had recently undergone high turnover; revising the security plan to include placing personnel to restrict access to scene areas; establishing additional cells to extend the range of the telephone system; revising the radio system for a greater range of operation; placing radios in more convenient areas; scheduling regular maintenance of radios to ensure that they are functioning at all times; having the fire department be responsible for transporting injured patients; and working with the sheriff and fire department to ensure better communication.[1]

Reference

1. Huser T.J.: Are your disaster plans ready, really ready? *J Healthc Prot Manage* 19(1):34–40, 2003.

Sidebar 10-4.
Conducting Exercises

Why does the standard require health care organizations (HCOs) to conduct regular emergency management exercises? And why does The Joint Commission stress the interaction of the organization and the community it serves as part of these exercises? The simple answer is that by conducting exercises, organizations test their ability to respond to emergencies. Exercises allow an organization to see the interaction of staff, supplies, equipment, and patients under the realistic scenarios the organization has designed based on what it knows about its own vulnerabilities. And if those scenarios sufficiently stress the organization's processes, the exercise reveals the strengths and weaknesses of the emergency operation plan (EOP) and leads to improvements.

Says Joe Cappiello, former Joint Commission vice president of Accreditation Field Operations, "In an uncertain world, performing effective drills are part of fulfilling your mission to the community and ensuring your survival as a health care entity." And, adds John Fishbeck, associate director, Division of Standards and Survey Methods, The Joint Commission, "Drilling offers an HCO the opportunity to form relationships with people in the community that it may need during a real emergency."

(continued)

Sidebar 10-4, *continued*

Conducting Exercises

Building on the Day-to-Day

No one could dispute the importance of preparedness, but designing and implementing good exercises requires time and energy. By nature, exercises are disruptive. But the impact of a real-time mass emergency on the organization and its community can be so overwhelming that the investment in drilling is well worth the effort. And that's precisely the point: to prepare leaders and staff to respond to significant disruptions.

Susan Goodwin, director, Quality Standards, Hospital Corporation of America (HCA), and a member of the Joint Commission's Committee on Healthcare Safety, fears that some facilities do not get that point: "HCOs need to go back to the EC standards and read the definition of *emergency*, which is, 'a natural or man-made event that *significantly disrupts* the environment of care or the organization's ability to provide care and treatment—or that significantly increases the demand for service.'"

In the most effective scenarios, Goodwin says, multiple systems should fail: "During the 9/11 response, hospitals reported that their water systems shut down. Also, air quality problems in New York disrupted ventilation systems. In real mass emergencies, the staff faces far more than a busy, stressful day."

On the other hand, say Cappiello and Fishbeck, HCOs already have an infrastructure for responding to unexpected events. "Joint Commission standards give guidance for dealing with daily emergencies," Cappiello says. "Because [HCO] staff know how to manage those incidents, we and they make assumptions that they are equipped to expand to large-scale events. Drilling is the proof of that assumption."

Fishbeck gives the example of staffing issues. All hospitals have staffing systems for codes—call lists and so on. In a drill or real mass emergency, they build on that basic structure. The same is true of supplies: They're needed every day, and every hospital has systems for ordering, tracking, and managing them. In an exercise, staff expand and flex that existing supply system.

Exploring the "What If" and the "How"

Constructing an effective exercise is a thinking process. It flows from the hazard vulnerability analysis (HVA) that organizations conduct to identify the emergencies they are most likely to face. Some are obvious—hurricanes in Florida, earthquakes in California. In most cases, natural disasters are higher-priority threats than terrorism. But, Goodwin cautions, an HVA should never be done in isolation. HCOs need lots of community input to identify the most pressing issues. And these issues shape the scenarios, as should the following guidelines.

Stress the System

Most HCOs have been exposed to short-term emergencies, lasting a few hours or days. Thus, their scenarios often address only immediate responses—for example, checking to see how many beds can be made available immediately or how many staff members can come in now. However, as Goodwin says, HCOs should plan as far as they can foresee—for weeks or even months of interrupted services.

"You might be able to get almost 100% of staff in for the immediate response, but what happens beyond that first day? How will you rotate staff? How will staff balance their professional responsibilities with their personal needs—for example, if they, too, have lost homes or loved ones?"

Executing the exercise means immersing everyone in the "how to" of responding to an emergency. And the "how to" lessons don't only come at the front end of the emergency (admissions). They focus on many other problems as well: how to get patients out of a facility; how to get employees, supplies, food, and water into it if the roads are jammed. Unless an exercise stresses the system, an HCO won't learn sufficient lessons.

(continued)

Sidebar 10-4, *continued*

Conducting Exercises

Goodwin suggests that planners play the "what if" game: "What if we had a hurricane and lost power for two weeks, our water was contaminated, our food suppliers couldn't get through, and our staff had their own personal troubles to deal with? What if we had thousands of dead bodies?"

Involve Multiple Levels

According to Judith Edwards, director of Emergency Preparedness for HCA and commander of a federal disaster medical assistance team, even since 9/11, many hospitals still haven't established adequate relationships with local, state, or federal emergency responders. Thus, scenarios should require participants to interact with others throughout the community—for example, working between alternative care sites, which encourages face-to-face interaction so that responders get to know each other. To stage an exercise of this magnitude, however, drill organizers must think creatively. Some use tabletop exercises, which are acceptable for the communitywide component of testing the EOP.

Set Specific Goals

Some organizations approach exercises with the goal of demonstrating how well their EOP works. However, Fishbeck and Cappiello caution, the real reward is finding out what you didn't know. It's discovering when, how, and why systems break down. Both Goodwin and Edwards emphasize the importance of going into an exercise knowing what you want to determine, and with specific goals for each department.

Says Edwards, "You may just focus on how you would move hundreds of patients through the system—from triage through discharge. Of course, that includes everything that goes with it: supplies, staff, transportation. Or a drill could emphasize decontamination, in which case you might be more concerned with equipment, training, and use of personal protective equipment." Or your exercise might focus on a total evacuation, in which case the crucial issues are where everyone would go (particularly if no other hospitals could take patients), how patients would be transported (particularly if no ambulances were available), and how staff would communicate between locations.

At one hospital where Edwards worked, the staff needed a smallpox response plan to prevent the spread of infection. Which doors would the infected patients use to enter the facility? Where would the infected patients be housed? Where would staff get extra supplies? Staff used the drill to answer their questions, to discover what worked and what didn't.

Test Multiple Aspects

An incident command system provides an organized response to an emergency—and a structure under which a facility's emergency plans can function—by designating responsibility and reporting relationships. Many hospitals are familiar with the Hospital Incident Command System (HICS) (formerly called the Hospital Emergency Incident Command System), which is focused on health care. HICS is flexible enough to fit organizations of all sizes and emergencies of all types, scopes, and time lines. It also provides a common vocabulary to ease coordination between emergency responders. Other models are available. The key is to discern how well the structure works in your community with various disaster scenarios.

Consider the following questions:

Is it flexible enough?
An all-hazards command structure—one that can apply to all scenarios—is preferable because it allows for flexibility and decision making during incidents.

(continued)

Sidebar 10-4, *continued*

Conducting Exercises

Does it provide a system for initiating and launching the emergency plan?
As Edwards explains, "Emergencies often happen on off-shifts, when administrators aren't there, so a nursing supervisor may have to make the determination about opening the command center." Some hospitals have a complexity analysis tool that allows a supervisor to score five areas and make a decision based on the composite score. The purpose is to assist personnel in determining whether the command center needs to be activated for any type of situation. "Activating a command center is expensive, so it's important to be able to justify the decision" notes Edwards.

Does it provide a system for notifying and coordinating the important players?
These include external authorities, such as local and state public health agencies, police and fire departments, and the Federal Emergency Management Agency, as well as hospital personnel.

Source: Adapted from Joint Commission Resources: How to conduct an EM drill. *Environment of Care News* 8:1, Jan. 2005.

Case Example: Mass Vaccination Drill Helps Organization Prepare for Possible Pandemic

Many scientists believe that it is just a matter of time before an influenza pandemic occurs. A pandemic can happen when the physical makeup of a virus changes and humans have no immunity to the altered virus. In that scenario, everyone could be vulnerable to the altered virus, and the consequences would be dire.[1] Unfortunately, the nature of biology is such that it's very hard, if not impossible, to predict if and when a pandemic could occur. The reality is that a virus could mutate tomorrow and become a pandemic virus, or it might never mutate. It's important that health care organizations and the communities they serve stay prepared and recognize that pandemics are as possible as earthquakes and hurricanes.[2]

In 2006 Kayenta Health Center participated in a mass vaccination drill to help fine-tune its pandemic response efforts. Kayenta Health Center, an ambulatory care facility, is a service unit in the Navajo Area Indian Health Service (NAIHS)—a division of the Department of Health and Human Services. NAIHS is responsible for the delivery of health services to Native Americans in portions of Arizona, New Mexico, Utah, and, to a lesser degree, Colorado. Kayenta Health Center's service area is spread across a remote and sparsely populated area and is in a traditional part of the Navajo reservation in northeast Arizona.

The idea to conduct a mass vaccination drill came from NAIHS, which required the service units within its jurisdiction to conduct such a drill on a specified day in November. Community members within the Navajo region were invited to participate and receive flu vaccinations at 11 service sites. The goal of the drill was to test how quickly and efficiently the different service units could vaccinate the entire community. To help its service units prepare, NAIHS created a template for a mass vaccination that each service unit could customize for its specific needs.

(continued)

Case Example: Mass Vaccination Drill Helps Organization Prepare for Possible Pandemic, *continued*

A Coordinated Effort

"Our organization uses the Hospital Incident Command System (HICS) and the National Incident Management System (NIMS) for emergency management," says Sherry Killingsworth, R.N., C.E.N., C.I.N.C., director of quality management, Kayenta Health Center. To prepare for its drill, Kayenta pulled together its incident commander; safety officer; public information officer; liaison officer; and planning, operations, logistics, communications, and finance chiefs (NIMS terminology) to begin discussions about how to structure the drill. The group convened weekly for planning sessions with local agencies and community members, including the fire and police departments. Within the planning sessions, each participant was assigned roles and responsibilities to be completed by the next planning session. The planning, operations, logistics, and communications chiefs met outside the weekly planning sessions with their assigned staff to ensure that adequate staffing, safety, supplies, and equipment were in place for the drill. The incident command team also met with the schools in the area to discuss their role in the pandemic drill.

Kayenta also communicated with other service units in the NAIHS region that were preparing for their mass vaccination drills. "We were able to participate in conference calls with these other sites and share information," says Killingsworth. "For example, the public information officer participated in conference calls with other public information officers to discuss how to effectively communicate the nature of the drill to the public and enlist their participation."

Addressing Snags Along the Way

As Kayenta was making final preparations for its drill, the organization ran into a problem. The local high school was designated through a memorandum of understanding (MOU) to be an alternative site for Kayenta Health Center in case of an emergency. Kayenta wanted to conduct its mass vaccination drill within this alternative site, to test how staff and the public would perform in a different location. "Usually when people want a flu shot, they come to the health center to get one. Staff and the public are familiar with the health center and the vaccination process there. We wanted to have the drill at a different site to test how staff and the public would function in an unfamiliar environment," says Killingsworth. Unfortunately, shortly before the designated date for the drill, the acting superintendent of the high school voiced concerns about using the high school as a designated alternative site. "We had to find an alternate location at the last minute," says Killingsworth. Kayenta met with the township and chapter (a Navajo Nation government entity), and they determined that the Kayenta Recreation Center—a boys' and girls' club—would be an appropriate location for the drill. "We needed a large space to conduct the drill because we were expecting more than 5,000 people to participate," says Killingsworth.

Another snag occurred when Killingsworth—the designated incident commander for Kayenta—became ill and was unable to fulfill her role. Kenneth Black, director of safety and security, for Kayenta, assumed the role of incident commander. "I was completely out of commission," says Killingsworth. "Ken stepped in and made a seamless transition to his new role."

Coping with a Mass Influx

Prior to the drill, Kayenta had requested that the local schools stagger the arrival of busloads of students to the recreation center to receive vaccinations. However, on the day of the drill, several busloads arrived at the same time, causing a mass influx of individuals into the site. "We had to restructure the flow to accommodate the mass influx. Although we didn't plan it that way, it did help test our capabilities to cope with a large number of individuals," says Black. "At our maximum throughput, we were vaccinating 1,200 people per hour."

(continued)

Case Example: Mass Vaccination Drill Helps Organization Prepare for Possible Pandemic, *continued*

Addressing Logistics

On the morning of the drill, all Kayenta staff reported to the recreation center at 5:00 A.M. to complete the setup for the drill, sign in, and receive assignments. The communications chief oversaw the setup of computers for patient registration, coding, and data entry. Drill evaluators were assigned to roam throughout the facility, monitoring and evaluating the drill. The drill lasted nine hours. During the course of the day, Kayenta vaccinated nearly 6,000 individuals.

Within the drill, Kayenta randomly designated 1 out of every 20 individuals entering the facility to be "sick" and proceed to the quarantine area for evaluation. "Also during the drill, we discovered some individuals who were actually sick or could become sick due to the vaccination. We quarantined those individuals as well," says Black. "We wanted to test our quarantine ability as well as our ability to distinguish between healthy and sick patients."

Learning from the Experience

A week after the drill, Kayenta held a debriefing in which it solicited feedback from external agencies as well as internal sources. After the debriefing, the incident command team, along with the planning, operations, logistics, communications, and finance chiefs, met and used information from the debriefing to create an executive summary of the event, which described what happened as well as what went well and what didn't. The summary also included an estimate of how much the drill cost, so that the organization could know the financial impact of a real mass vaccination situation.

One of the biggest lessons Kayenta learned in the course of the drill was the importance of emergency management training. "During the drill, we realized that not every organization leader participating in the drill had experienced HICS or NIMS training, so they were not familiar with how those systems worked. It would have been helpful if everyone had been trained on HICS and NIMS so that they could have understood more quickly their role in the emergency management process," says Killingsworth.

Kayenta also learned the importance of communication. "Because of our location, cell phone usage is spotty. Radio communication and phone lines were also limited in outlying areas. We found it difficult to inform people in some locations about the drill. We used pagers and messengers but plan to improve communication infrastructure in the near future," says Black.

Kayenta planned to use the lessons learned from this drill in its next scheduled drill to improve its emergency response efforts. Likewise, it planned to use the successes achieved in the mass vaccination drill to help frame subsequent drills.

References

1. Gellin B.: *How Do Pandemic Viruses Occur?* Centers for Disease Control and Prevention. http://www.pandemicflu.gov/news/transcripts/question1070.html (accessed Apr. 17, 2007).
2. Agwunobi J.: *Will a Pandemic Virus Occur?* Centers for Disease Control and Prevention. http://www.pandemic flu.gov/news/transcripts/question1071.html (accessed Apr. 17, 2007).

Source: Reprinted from Joint Commission Resources: Conducting a mass vaccination drill. *Environment of Care News* 10:7, Jul. 2007.

For Additional Assistance

The Agency for Healthcare Quality and Research (AHRQ) has released a tool designed to evaluate hospital disaster exercises using evaluation modules and addenda. The modules assess the incident command, decontamination, triage, and treatment zones.

The zone modules address time points, zone description, personnel, zone operations, communication, information flow, security, victim documentation and tracking, victim flow, personal protective equipment and safety, equipment and supplies, staff rotation, and zone disruption. The tool also includes a module for per-exercise assessment and debriefing. The addenda address biological incidents, radiological incidents, general observation and documentation, and victim tracking. *The Evaluation of Hospital Disaster Drills: A Module-Based Approach,* which was designed by the Johns Hopkins University Evidence-Based Practice Center, can be downloaded from AHRQ's Web site at http://www.ahrq.gov/research/hospdrills/hospdrill.htm.

Other resources for additional assistance include the following:

- Disaster Planning Drills and Readiness Assessment, AHRQ: http://www.ahrq.gov/news/ulp/btbriefs/btbrief2.htm
- Bioterrorism Tabletop Exercise, National Association of County & City Health Officials: http://www.nacchol.org/bttoolbox
- Disaster Preparedness Exercise Development and Design Guidance from New England, Northern New England Metropolitan Medical Response System: http://www.nnemmrs.org/exercises.html

References

1. Joint Commission Resources: *Safer Emergency Care: Strategies and Solutions.* Oakbrook Terrace, IL: Joint Commission on Accreditation of Healthcare Organizations, 2007.
2. Joint Commission Resources: *Infection Control Issues in the Environment of Care.* Oakbrook Terrace, IL: Joint Commission on Accreditation of Healthcare Organizations, 2005.

Index

D

E

M

N

O

P

T

U

V

W